A

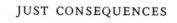
JUST CONSEQUENCES

'In nature there are neither rewards nor punishments – there are consequences.'

Robert E. Ingersoll, *Lectures and Essays.*

JUST CONSEQUENCES

A survey of some contemporary health problems in relation
to nutrition which suggests that there is a new pattern of
diseases in Western civilisation.

A symposium edited by
ROBERT WALLER

CHARLES KNIGHT & CO. LTD.
LONDON
1971

Charles Knight & Co. Ltd.,
11/12 Bury Street, London EC3A 5AP,
Dowgate Works, Douglas Road, Tonbridge, Kent.

First published 1971

SBN 85314 105 3

Printed in Great Britain by Lewis Reprints Ltd.
A member of the Brown Knight & Truscott group.

To

Jack and Mary Pye

for their generous contributions to nutritional research

Contents

Contents

1. Introduction
A new pattern of diseases in
western civilisation

Robert Waller

Robert Waller, editor of the Journal of the Soil Association, is the biographer of Sir George Stapledon, who was the founder of the Welsh Plant Breeding Station and an agrarian philosopher. Mr Waller edited his posthumous book 'Human Ecology'.

IN an age of human ecology we must draw together the threads both of our civilisation and culture and examine their relationship to each other. The contributors to this symposium have related our contemporary diet to a new pattern of western diseases. They have also indicated how our diet is interwoven with our industrial technology and way of life.

At the beginning of our century there was widespread optimism about the benefits to be expected from the application of science to medical problems. The savage, lethal epidemics seemed to be under control. A steady material improvement in the living conditions of the mass of the people had far-reaching effects on the incidence of disease. From 1839 until 1870, the crude annual death rate was 25-30 per thousand living; after 1870 the death rate fell steadily until by 1921 it was 12 per thousand living. We have to remember, too, that despite the horrors of the working conditions in the factories, it was these factories that made possible the increase in the birth rate and produced the goods which were slowly to improve material conditions, as well as to stunt the individual lives of the

1

work people and spread pollution. Since 1921, however, in spite of the great advances in medical treatment and conditions of work, the death rate has fallen very slowly indeed. The crude death rate for heart disease rose from 1,500 per million in 1895 to 3,750 per million in 1955. And for cancer in the same period the figure rose from 800 to nearly 2,000 per million and is reaching epidemic proportions.

In America during the last decades the lengthening of life expectancy has ground almost to a halt and is lower than in England and Wales. In the life expectancy table (males 1963) England and Wales came tenth with 68.0 years, while the U.S. was twenty-first with 66.6, although it is the richest country in the world. Something is evidently going wrong with progress.

The antibiotic era that began in 1935 undoubtedly benefitted the young who, says Dr. Deryck Taverner in *The Impending Medical Revolution* 'survived to develop the almost inevitable degenerative and malignant conditions that we have so far either failed to prevent or to cure to any significant extent.' This symposium deals with that problem, convinced on the evidence that these diseases are not inevitable but are caused largely by the kind of food that we eat.

The mortality per thousand aged 25-34 years fell from 1.75 in 1949 to 1.07 in 1962. In the age group 45-53 years the death rate fell from 8.39 to 7.25 in the same period. Dr. Taverner comments, 'nevertheless, it is hard to escape from the conclusion that the great advances in medical science in the last century have mainly resulted in a change in the patterns and age incidence of disease. Disease now seldom kills or maims the young. Instead they survive to suffer the manifold diseases of old age long before they kill.' Our contributors agree with that: but they also believe they can help to explain it.

The increasing number of old people in Europe and America derives from greater survival among the young and middle aged. In general, though, people over the age of fifty live very little longer than their grandparents. The expectation of life for a man of fifty in 1841 was 20 years: in 1967 it was 23 years. Not a very startling difference. Dr. Hugh Sinclair has dealt with this historically in his paper on page 85.

Many medical writers are depressed by the immense expenditure on health services that has failed to cope with the diseases of the second half of life. How serious these are has been summed up in a paper given to the Royal Society of Health in April, 1967, entitled *Health Hazards in Middle Age – Statistics of the Risks.* Dr. R. Logan, Director of the Medical Care Research Unit, Manchester University, summarised these hazards as follows:

For men: 1 in 4 will suffer from chronic bronchitis
1 in 5 will develop coronary heart disease
1 in 12 will have a peptic ulcer
1 in 4 will develop cancer, of which
1 in 30 will be cancer of the lung
1 in 12 will be admitted to a general hospital each year
1 in 300 will be admitted to a psychiatric hospital each year.

For women: 1 in 4 will be regularly attending a GP with a chronic disease
1 in 8 will die of diabetes
1 in 5 will develop cancer, of which
1 in 20 will die of cancer of the breast
1 in 14 will be admitted to a general hospital each year
1 in 200 will be admitted to a psychiatric hospital each year.

Dr. Logan also says that sickness absence has doubled since the last war and that of men in their early fifties 5% are incapacitated through illness and the rate accelerates in the early sixties to 13%

Is it right to accept the view that these degenerative diseases are only due to failure to cope with conditions

3

that have always existed but with which we have so far failed to come to grips in the way that we have done with the infectious diseases? The experience of the doctors and surgeons writing in this symposium suggests that this is not the case and that we are dealing with a new phenomenon. They base this conclusion on the comparison of the patterns of disease in western nations with those in less technologically developed nations.

When he was senior surgeon at the Radcliffe Infirmary, Oxford, Mr. Elliot-Smith studied the hospital records and discovered that there were only 5 cases of appendicitis between 1895 and 1905. There are now over 500 cases in this hospital every year. Stomach ulcers were not recorded before the 1890s. Yet in the last war 23,500 were discharged from the army with ulcers over a period of 30 months (1939-1941). These ulcers were not due to army life or army cooking: most of the recruits brought their ulcers with them. When Mr. Elliot-Smith examined the records of six separate London hospitals from 1925-1929, a dramatic rise in ulcers was revealed even over this short period.

Like Mr. Knights and Surgeon-Captain Cleave – two other surgeons contributing to this symposium – Elliot-Smith had worked in Africa and like them he had noted that among those native peoples who did not eat western foods, there was an absence of the diseases most prevalent in this country. It was this that led him to search the hospital records to find out if these diseases were newcomers or if they had always been present. His conclusions are in his paper on page 143. In his search for explanations, he encountered other doctors, surgeons and research workers, many of them contributors to this book, whose similar experiences had set them on the same trail. In 1969 the Soil Association invited some of them to contribute to its Annual Conference at Attingham Park. This symposium is based on the papers given there: additional papers have been contributed by those who were unable to come. Since the Soil Association's aim is to investigate the relationships between soil, plant, animal, man and health, this theme fits into its own educational work and research. The second half of this book is concerned with the Association's research into the relationship between diet and health.

Surgeon-Captain Cleave also confirmed that Africans who ate western food developed the new western diseases, while those who were still eating their traditional food did not. A comparison of the hospital records in western food areas with those in less technologically advanced areas revealed that the western diseases included far more than appendicitis and ulcers: they extended to diabetes, obesity, coronary thrombosis, dental decay, varicose veins, diverticulitis, constipation and several infections of the bowels probably related to constipation.

The most obvious difference in the diet between the two groups is that the western diet has white sugar and white bread, processed, packaged and synthetic, while the older peasant diets are based on unrefined cereals, fruit and sugar – what we now call 'wholefood'. Little or nothing has been removed from the sugar cane and the grain.

Cleave and his collaborators found that as the consumption of white flour and white sugar increased, so did the new diseases. In war time, when these refined foods were rationed and/or the extraction of nutrients and bran from bread had been limited by law, then these diseases declined, only to shoot up again when the restraints were removed. Today we eat as much as 10 times more sugar per head per annum than did our forbears at the end of the 18th century.

Since carbohydrates are broken down to sugar in the body, it is useful to give the diseases to which sugar contributes one name: for this reason Cleave groups the diseases just listed under one name – the saccharine disease. Mr. Denis P. Burkitt of the Medical Research Council has suggested, in a recent paper on the saccharine disease *(The Lancet*, 6.12.69) that cancer of the colon may be implicated. Food, he writes, takes six to eight times longer to pass through the intestines of those living in western countries than in parts of Africa and India. 'I know of no country where the rarity in incidence of bowel cancer and diverticular disease are not associated, and there is experimental evidence suggesting a relationship of the latter to diet.' Mr. Burkitt believes that research should be done on the relation between the rate of bowel flow and intestinal diseases. He concludes his paper:

'If a relationship can be established between dietary habits and disease patterns it should not be necessary to wait for an understanding of the mechanism whereby benign or malignant disease is produced before attempting prevention.' By the time we have established 'proof' many thousands more people will have died unnecessarily.

Dr. Hugh Sinclair would also incriminate some animal fats. He illustrates his argument with a new example – lung cancer. Lung cancer is now associated with smoking: but in Spain and Japan where smoking is as common as in our country, lung cancer hardly exists. So there must be another factor, Dr. Sinclair believes that he has tracked it down to the saturated fatty acids in animal fats.

The membranes of the cells of our bodies are strengthened by the incorporation of fatty acids. The unsaturated *essential* fatty acids are not made by the body and have to be taken in through food. There are also *non-essential* saturated fatty acids which do not serve the same essential function when assimilated by the membranes of the cells.

The essential fatty acids tend to be unstable in air and turn rancid, so the manufacturers have found a means of changing their chemistry by saturating them; this process hardens the originally soft fat.

The membranes of the cells of our bodies serve to protect the cells from invasion and penetration by alien bodies likely to damage them. If the membranes are weakened by poor nutrition their defensive function is weakened and they become more permeable and are therefore more likely to be injured by foreign substances of all kinds, including cigarette smoke.

Dr. Sinclair's experiments with pigs have shown that under natural conditions they tend to produce soft fats. Under modern indoor conditions pigs are fed, however, so

6

as to produce hard fat which is easier for the meat trade to handle.* These hard fats, deficient in the essential fatty acids, play a large part in our diet and may cause increased permeability of the body cells, a phenomenon frequently observed today in western countries. Obviously this could contribute to many different diseases, including the saccharine disease.

Dr. Sinclair advances statistical and historical evidence to support his clinical experience and his animal feeding experiments. He points to the rise in chronic heart disease – which he particularly associates with the saturated fatty acids – and lung cancer in 1943, when three foodstuffs arrived from America – hydrogenated margarine (i.e. with the fatty acids saturated), very fat bacon and tinned meat that is rich in saturated fat. These, through Lend-Lease, introduced a great increase of non-essential fatty acids into our food which are taken up into the cell membranes in the place of essential fatty acids. Here they act like ill-fitting bricks within the metabolic and bio-chemical cell structures. Dr. Sinclair has described some ingenious studies carried out during the war in mental hospitals in Scandinavia. The patients were schizoid and unaware that a war was going on: so the stress factor was constant and not increased by the war. Two different groups of patients were fed carefully controlled diets and the conclusion was that saturated fatty acids increased the tendency to coronary thrombosis.

Evidence relating changes of living conditions to disease is described by Dr. Innes Pearse in her paper on page 63. Harry Walters found that animals removed from their natural surroundings to a life indoors developed dietary deficiency diseases and anaemia, the diseases prevalent in the early days of the industrial revolution.

In our symposium we show that the nutritional theories implied by the way we eat and feed our crops in farming are over-simplified. Michael Blake[2] demonstrates that the

*This was supported by Michael Crawford, Nuffield Institute of Medicine, in a long letter to *The Lancet* (27.12.70).

concentrated fertilisers (especially the high ratio nitrogen fertilisers) that we use in agriculture today only supply three nutrients (NPK – nitrogen, phosphate and potassium) while the plant must take up many more than these from the soil. This refinement of our plant foods is similar to the refinement of flour and sugar in our own diet: not only does it result in a deficiency of essential minerals and nutrients but it over-concentrates the substances that are not abstracted. In the cycles of nature the nutrients taken up by the plant are returned in the process of decomposition: but when fertilisers are substituted man makes the decision as to which nutrients will be returned and his knowledge of the subject is not sufficient to justify him in doing this. Obviously in time our soils must become deficient in reserves of essential nutrients. As farm animals as well as ourselves have to eat the produce of these deficient soils, diseases related to these deficiencies will follow. Soil structure is also involved. A good soil structure – one which drains well and allows the passage of air to the roots of the plants – depends upon the activity of many inhabitants of the soil striving to create the best living conditions for themselves: this competitive work plays a fundamental part in creating the architecture of the soil. And these workers have to be fed. A deficiency of humus in the soil, resulting from reliance upon fertilisers, also contributes to the general breakdown of soil life. It is a complex picture surveyed in considerable detail by Cmdr. Blake (page 34) with its practical implications. At the time of writing a government report on soil structure has just been published which admits that soil structures in many parts of the country have seriously deteriorated and that lack of money prevents the farmer from practising good husbandry. Research at Haughley has shown the effect on soil structure of farming by three different methods of land use. The difference is quite dramatic and points to the dangers of monocultural cereal growing and the need to return to rotations and mixed farming. For economic reasons this is unpopular with governments. But it is ecology and not economics that is the ultimate necessity, as Sir George Stapledon never tired of trying to tell the officials of his own day.

In this symposium we mount four dimensions of attack on this problem of the new diseases: evidence from hospital records over a hundred years: comparisons of diet and disease in different areas of the world: animal feeding experiments (Trevor McSheehy's paper on page 151) and the treatment of soil and plant in modern husbandry. We conclude that the diseases are just consequences of a disregard for fundamental principles of nature.

For too long our health and our food have been kept in separate departments: one under the Ministry of Agriculture, Fisheries and Food, the other under the Ministry of Health. Surely the extravagant use of pesticides and herbicides and antibiotics would never have been allowed if medical research had been allowed more say? Surely it is more important that food should be a means of creating a healthy nation than that it should be grown primarily simply to make a profit? Yet successive governments by their policies have forced farmers to model their husbandry on the principles of mass production industry: this, in the long run, is not possible: the farmers' raw material is biological, not inorganic. The effort to enforce this on a large scale can bring about a crisis in civilisation, similar to that which destroyed the Romans, whose agriculture was wrecked as the small farmer was ousted by the great landed estates growing wheat year after year. Even the new Department of the Environment, clearly a good reform in itself, has excluded the Ministries of Agriculture and Health. Yet our main anxiety about the pollution of the environment must be the effects on the health of man. I mention this to show the inadequacy of our conception of the problem that confronts us. The degradation of the quality of food through the misuse of technology is a form of environmental contamination.

A few farsighted thinkers – Sir Charles Galton Darwin in *The Next Million Years* (1953), Dr. Hugh Nicol in *The Limits of Man* (1969)[3] – have pointed out that in the long run nature will be protected against the exploitive powers of man when the fossil fuels required to provide the energy for our industrial civilisation are exhausted. At the present rate at which we are using up our oil – and this rate is always increasing – it is unlikely to last for more than a hundred years and one authoritative source predicts only 37 years. How few people realise that the high yields of modern farming depend upon energy brought on to the farm from outside? Five tons of oil are required to produce one ton of nitrogen fertiliser. The tractors with which we do our cultivations (and which put stress upon our degraded soil structures) require fuel. This fuel is nature's capital, not the interest. What happens when this capital is exhausted?

Good husbandry is the model of how to maintain production without using up capital. The aim of good husbandry is to intensify the renewable energies of nature (as by renewing nitrogen through clover and other legumes). Chiefly this means working with the biological cycle. The first half of this cycle is the growth half which results in the saleable product, the second half is the process of biodegradation or decomposition which feeds the soil with the waste products of the crop. So far as man is concerned this is uneconomic. Animal manures, the residues of animal metabolism, are similarly regarded as an unprofitable nuisance, an example of inefficiency on the part of nature. Yet the full cycle is absolutely essential to biological survival. But this over-simplification of natural processes for the sake of fitting into our economic system cannot last. As soon as the energy which man mines from nature is finished, he is back again in the traditional situation in which he must renew energy in the way that nature does it, through the plant, or by the utilisation of wind and water. This is why research into organic farming, which is not dependent upon chemicals and fertilisers, is so important for the future of our food supplies, apart from many other good reasons related to health and flavour.

The abnormal conditions of the 19th century – when

our population quadrupled and we were able to feed it from the soils of the new world and by the ingenuities of technology dependent upon fossil fuels – masked from us the temporary nature of our wealth. And yet we termed the wealth progress and assumed that the means of providing it was infinite. The looming crisis of energy will amount to a revolution in thought, in ways of life and in political ideas: a revolution which will be the reverse of the industrial revolution. Deep in ourselves we know this to be true and, in order to save ourselves, we blind ourselves and frenetically intensify those very policies that are going to bankrupt us. A thrifty husbanding of the resources of nature, especially the capital-energy resources, is our only hope. Respect for the relationship between man and nature is the first principle of human ecology. Our civilisation is inhuman because it ignores this.

Although we think of ourselves as a scientific civilisation, this is not strictly true for we do not accept the discipline of science. We have made it the handmaiden of technology. The fundamental principles of science indicate we are heading for disaster as clearly as the laws of thermodynamics showed that perpetual motion was not possible. It was not until engineers accepted this discipline based upon scientific understanding that the construction of efficient machines was possible. It is always best to work within the limitations imposed by nature and it is science that teaches us, in the material sphere, what these are. These limits impose a discipline upon man's anarchic appetites now harnessed to technology and industry. Indeed the attempt to accept discipline is treated as cowardly by those whose power determines the course of our society. The revolt of the young is based upon their scorn for the uncontrolled violence and greed of their elders in the field of economics. They do not, as the older generation does, take our civilisation for granted and we are angry. But they are right, even though they have not yet understood in practical detail what is wrong. We cannot take for granted a civilisation based upon illusions.

11

This is not a digression from the main theme of this symposium. All our contributors point out the need to accept the discipline of nature as revealed to us by science itself, real science – not the science that is stifled when it runs contrary to the needs and ambitions of economists and industrialists and politicians and those scientists who are their harlots. The present is haunted by the realisation that the future will be different to what we anticipated: that to adjust ourselves to it will mean a major re-evaluation of every dimension of life, a total human response.

Finally let us return to the main theme of this symposium as we encounter it now and ask ourselves what we can do. Our contributors show that the degenerative diseases resulting from a degradation of our diet is shortening the expectation of life after middle age. Our bodies will sustain a lot of ill-treatment before they can no longer sustain a working life. Nature is surprisingly tolerant of abuse and it is this that tempts us into fatal efforts to outwit her. Doctors refer to the twenty years' abuse, meaning that we can abuse our natural health for twenty years or so before the effects begin to show: which brings us up to the age of about forty-five. It is from then onwards that the statistics show that the modern diseases strike.

The rules of good health – fresh air, fresh food, adequate exercise and a temperate attitude of mind – have been handed down from generation to generation in a perennial philosophy for those ready to listen. The tragedy of today is that many advances in technology – successful in realising the aims set them by industry – are placing these conditions of good health out of reach of most citizens. We are becoming aware of the dangers of contamination by atomic radiation, toxic sprays, fertiliser run-off into surface waters, sewage disposal into lakes, rivers and seas, car exhausts, diesel fumes and industrial wastes generally through the oxidation of fossil fuels. Threatening as these are, the evidence presented in this book indicates that changes in the composition of our food, arising from technological skill, also play a lethal part in this degeneration of health dramatically revealed in the second half of life.

At our Conference at Attingham on this theme, the chairman, Harry Walters, summing up, said: How does one look at all this? It would seem clear that we have high-lighted several main factors:

1. That over-intake of harmful fats, refined sugar and flour and over-processed foods is clinically dangerous.
2. That more effort should be made to communicate these dangers to the public.
3. That in eating balanced diets of organically produced foods these dangers are substantially reduced.
4. That farming should not ideally be regarded as a mass production industry and that the policies of the Ministries of Health and Agriculture should be aligned more to serve the health of the people.
5. In every country organic farms should be maintained to provide those long term controls which will assure the continuance of optimal soil structure and fertility.
6. That modern man urgently needs an overall biophilo-sophy to link the technical age to ancient wisdom.

References
1. The statistics relating to England and Wales are taken from Dr. Taverner's *The Impending Medical Revolution* (Hodder & Stoughton, 1968.) The American figures from *The Coming Revolution in Medicine* by Dr. David D. Rutstein (M.I.T. Press, 1967).
2. Both Cmdr. Blake and Surgeon-Captain Cleave refer to their published work in their articles.
3. *The Limits of Man,* Dr. Hugh Nicol (Constable, 1969). *The Next Million Years,* Sir Charles Galton Darwin (Rupert Hart Davis, 1953).

The fossil fuel situation in relation to our future has been summed up by Hugh Nicol in the following extract from a talk he gave to the Attingham Soil Association Annual Conference, 1970:

'All life depends on the behaviour of water and its elements – oxygen for oxidation and every sort of burning, including consuming food: hydrogen for the converses (producing more food). There cannot be one of these without the other.

Pollution arises in every instance by making oxygen combine with fossil fuels. Causing hydrogen to combine with nitrogen and sulphur and to produce food (animal energy) is done either by burning fossil fuel to make fertilisers and to power agricultural machines, etc., or by relying on photosynthesis plus the inherent chemistry of the soil. The latter alternative limits population to what it was a couple of centuries ago.

Since the present population is much greater than what surface resources can keep alive, and is using up fossil resources intensively for 'amenity' or hedonistic purposes which have no relation to food, the alternatives are plain; and because the population must ultimately fall, we can talk about *'fertility' (of people or crops) only for a limited future:* that is, for as long as fossil fuel is everywhere abundant.

Man is the only animal who has made fossil fuels, and their products, part of his environment. The choices henceforth are roughly: Will you prefer to be choked, run down by a machine, or starve?'

The urgency of the need to cope with the degenerative diseases and the probability that they will lead to a breakdown of the medical services is pointed out by Dr. Taverner in the book already cited. He estimates that at the present day scale of 10 beds per thousand population, we shall have to build, commission and staff a new 600 bedded general hospital every three months just to keep up with the load of the next thirty-five years. But in the last thirty-five years we have only built fifteen new general hospitals in the whole country. So at the same time we shall be forced to replace our existing stock of hospitals as well. To deal with this situation we should need to provide two new general hospitals every month from now until the year 2000. Prevention is better than bankruptcy?

2. The conception of the Saccharine Disease: an outline

T.L. Cleave, M.R.C.P. (Lond.), Surgeon-Captain, R.N. (retired)

Formerly Director of Medical Research, R.N. Medical School, Captain Cleave is joint author with Dr. G.D. Campbell and Mr. N.S. Painter of 'Diabetes, Coronary Thrombosis and the Saccharine Disease.' Like the other medical contributors to this book, who have all worked in countries where western diets are not eaten, he believes that the so-called diseases of civilisation are chiefly due to refined sugar and flour.

Part I. Conditions Involved

IN a paper in 1956[1] I advanced the hypothesis that many, if not most, of the modern degenerative diseases could be ascribed to a single cause – the refining of carbohydrates, and especially to the refining of sugar, with its enormous subsequent rise in consumption over a century and a half. The conditions and their modes of production were set out, and, in a later work, on peptic ulcer[2], the conditions were classified in accordance with these modes of production, and the central disease of which they were considered the manifestations was termed the Saccharine Disease.

The word saccharine (which, following the Oxford English Dictionary, is pronounced like the river Rhine, to separate it sharply from the chemical sweetener) means related to sugar. It is true that in the production of this disease I unquestionably include the refining of starch, as in the refining of various grains and (in the tropics) of manioc, but as starch ends up in the body as sugar

15

(glucose), the term saccharine disease seemed more convenient than heavier alternatives. It still does.

The main conditions set out, with their modes of production were the following.

From over-consumption:
Diabetes
Obesity
Coronary thrombosis
Primary B.coli infections (appendicitis, cholesystitis, etc.)

From the removal of fibre:
Dental caries and periodental disease. ('pyorrhoea')
Colonic stasis, with its complications of varicose veins, femoral thrombosis and haemorrhoids, and of diverticulitis (or, as stated more accurately in a later, joint work[3]: diverticulosis preceding diverticulitis).

From the removal of protein:
Peptic ulcer

It is particularly to be noted that the concentration in the carbohydrates has been produced, not by the removal of water, but by the removal of fibre (and of protein), so the conditions produced by over-consumption automatically predispose to the conditions produced by the removal of fibre (and of protein). For this reason the term 'saccharine disease', which is really only applicable to the first group, is not as unsuitable as it appears – and the convenience remains. It is also a fact that all these disease conditions stem from a single motive – to get at the main nutrients in the carbohydrate foods and reject the accompanying fibre.

Other conditions were also alluded to, such as renal calculus, from the alteration produced in the reaction of the urine, and I have no doubt whatever that in the years to come other workers will add other conditions, together with their modes of production.

The list already seems a long one and it might well be asked whether attributing so many conditions to the same cause might not point to loss of perspective. But I hold the exact opposite view. For it would be a coincidence indeed if these refined carbohydrates, which are known to produce havoc on the teeth, did not also have profound repercussions on other parts of the alimentary canal during their passage along it, and on other parts of the body after absorption from the canal. How many diseases for that matter involve but one system? One need only point, for example, to the systematic manifestations of syphilis, ranging from insanity to aneurysm, to see that no loss of perspective need be present in the conception now under consideration.

Part II. Hereditary Defects and Personal Builds

Before alluding to the conditions themselves it is necessary to make some preliminary observations. First of all, the conception of the saccharine disease is based strictly on the Darwinian theory, so that the human body, after many millions of years of evolutionary adaptation, is regarded as correctly constructed, and its breakdown in the above conditions as due to exposing it to one or more new environmental factors to which it cannot yet possibly be adapted. In short, and in plain English, the body in these conditions is regarded 'as built rightly but as being used wrongly' – an exoteric phrase redeemed by its clarity.

It is true that an exception to the body being built correctly exists in the case of congenital defects, such as hare lip, but even under the protection of modern civilisation such defects never exceed the figure of 5 per 1,000 births[4] – a frequency only one-twentieth of many of the conditions enumerated above. This crucial difference in frequency demonstrates the weakness in ascribing such conditions to congenital defect, a weakness which is clinched by the very recent appearance of these conditions in the time-scale, and by their rarity in races still living under primitive conditions, as will be shown later.

At this point must be considered the totally different

17

question of 'personal build'. For a man's personal build, absolutely healthy though it normally is, may render him highly vulnerable to a new environmental factor. In a monograph on varicose veins[5], which was an extension of the above paper, I used a simile of tall men in warfare being especially vulnerable to machine-gun-fire; and similar variations in personal build, *which involve every structure in the body*, readily explain why certain persons suffer from a disease produced by a new environmental factor whereas other persons do not. For example, as regards varicose veins, which the present conception ascribes to pressure on the external iliac veins by an unnaturally loaded colon, from a refined diet, the relationship of one man's colon to the iliac veins may be quite different from another man's, and thus his vulnerability in this respect may be quite different, too. And it is easy to see the fundamental difference between a disease produced by a perfectly healthy build, that happens to be vulnerable to a new factor in the environment, and a disease based on congenital defect. The distinction is crucial, because in the personal-build case the basic external cause of the disease can be removed at once, whereas in the congenital-defect case the cause can never be removed, though it may be remedied. For this reason I prefer the term personal build to genetic susceptibility, which latter term carries an atmosphere of defect.

Hereditary Features Deceptive

It can now be seen how deceptive hereditary features in disease can be, *for personal build is just as hereditary as congenital defect*. A tall man killed by machine-gun-fire in World War I could have had a tall son killed by machine-gun-fire in World War II. In my opinion, hereditary features in diseases like those enumerated above concern vulnerable personal builds and *not* congenital defects, and can therefore be virtually disregarded. I believe that at the present much time and energy are being devoted to hereditary features that are nothing less than a snare and a delusion.

18

It would seem far wiser to regard the body 'as built rightly but as being used wrongly,' and aim at removing the causative unnatural from the environment.

I make no apology for using plain rather than academic English in the above paragraphs, for only too often at the present time does the body appear to be made at fault over disease when it should not be, and only too seldom does there appear to be appreciated the deep pitfall lying behind any hereditary features present.

Part III. The Refining of Carbohydrates

Against this most essential background there is now presented in outline the new environmental factor constituted by the refining of flour and sugar, and the following chart summarises the position as regards refined sugar (which includes both white and brown sugar):

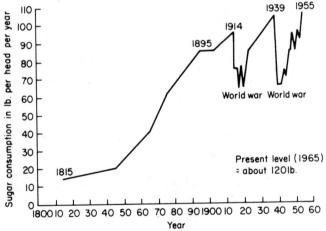

Fig. 1.—The rise in sugar consumption in the United Kingdom over the last century and a half. (*Drawn from information kindly supplied by Fairrie & Co. and the 'Board of Trade Journal'.*)

It will be seen in the round that the 15lb. of sugar consumed per head per year in 1815 have jumped in only 150 years to the 8-fold figure of 120lb. in 1965. The latter figure equals a daily consumption of about 5oz. per person

– which is the amount of sugar contained in some 2½lb. of sugar beet. And it is precisely this unnatural concentration in the sugar, through which 2½lb. of sugar beet loses its fibre and gives place to 5oz. of neat sugar, that exemplifies the new environmental factors we have been discussing, and that, deceiving both appetite and satiety, leads to startling increases in consumption. For who on the same diet could replace his sugar intake by 2½lb. of sugar beet?

Refining of Flour

Turning now to the case of flour, it may be said that in the refining of wheat, which dates on a massive scale from only about 200 years ago, approximately a third of the grain is stripped off and discarded – and this third is the one that contains much of the protein and nearly all the fibre, the importance of which will be seen later. The concentration produced is less than in the case of sugar, but is nevertheless easily revealed in the eating (e.g. solid wholemeal bread versus puffy white bread). It is true that there has been a fall in bread consumption in recent times, but this is largely due to the more serious rise in sugar consumption, and does not alter the crucial fact that present bread consumption is greater than it would be if the missing third of fibre (bran) were returned to the bread that is still eaten*.

The serious consequences of refining wheat and other grains are perhaps more clearly revealed in the East (e.g. in the ulcer-belt of India), where the consumption of polished rice is not accompanied by any large consumption of sugar, but it can also be revealed in this country by the dramatic shortening of the bowel transit-time when the removed bran is restored to the diet, of which more later.

Now the starch in white flour is digested to, and is absorbed as, sugar (glucose). The same is largely true of the ordinary white and brown sugar sold in grocers' shops; any slight qualitative differences, being natural, need not detain us in this outline. But the *quantitative* differences are important, the sugar having been rendered more con-

*The main refining of flour took place in the 18th century and that of sugar in the 19th century. The roller-milling of flour introduced about 1880 produced a whiter flour, but removed little extra fibre (bran), since most of this is removed in the lighter degrees of milling.

centrated than the starch, and hence rendered still more dangerous. With this significant proviso, therefore, no great distinction will be made here between the consumption of refined (white) flour and refined sugar, as regards their effects on the human body.

Fats

Lastly, the saccharine conception concerns itself very little with fat consumption. It is true that some fats, such as butter and vegetable oils, have been concentrated by man to much the same extent as have the carbohydrates, but the concentration here never seems to deceive either the appetite or satiety. I believe the reason for this is that such fats do not reach, let alone exceed, the concentration present in many natural fats. For example, whereas butter and margarine contain about 85% of fat, the perinephric fat (suet) in oxen and sheep contains some 99% of fat. The Jack Sprats who desire no fat, and their wives who desire a great deal of fat, can therefore still follow their natural instincts effectively today. In close accord with this, the increase in fat consumption in recent times has been only a small fraction of the increase in sugar consumption noted above. And to maintain that saturated animal fats, such as occur in butter and in our native roast beef, are bad for us, whereas unsaturated fats like sunflower seed oil are good for us, would make us, evolutionarily, not men, but something akin to a flock of greenfinches – and it is not surprising that no benefit has ever been proved to follow the substitution of the ones for the others. Also, the variations in the levels of the blood lipids, of which so much has been made, is well recognised today as being related to carbohydrate consumption as well as to fat consumption.

We now pass to the study of the conditions themselves, as set out in the above list, but proceeding this time in anatomical sequence.

Part IV. The Manifestations of the Saccharine Disease

Dental Conditions

Starting in the mouth, the loss of the cleansing power of the fibre in unrefined carbohydrates on the teeth, and the loss of the stimulating power of this fibre on the gums, is too well known as the dominant factor in Dental Decay, and in the equally serious Periodental Disease ('pyorrhoea'), to need much discussion here. Reference, however, may be made to the late Professor A. B. MacGregor's survey in Ghana in 1964[8], which showed how directly the incidence of these conditions varied with the deviation of the diet from unrefined to refined carbohydrates; and to Professor J. L. Hardwick's work[9]; showing how the rise in the caries rate over the centuries has accompanied first the refining of flour and later the refining of sugar also.

Peptic Ulcer

Turning now to the next site of impact of these refined carbohydrates, the stomach, I have with much labour accumulated a large mass of evidence incriminating these foods as the essential cause of *gastric* and *duodenal ulcer*[2]. In that work I reject unequivocally that the cause of these conditions ever lies in the body being at fault, either in 'acid attack' or in 'mucosal defence', and argue, instead, that the cause lies essentially in the partial or complete removal of the protein component of carbohydrate foods. Protein, be it remembered, is the *only* food material that neutralises the gastric acid, and in the refining of carbohydrates the protein is removed to an extent that varies from 12% in the refining of wheat to 100% in the refining of sugar-beet or sugar-cane. The resulting loss of buffering power has been measured[10], and the consequent faster climb in the acid curve in test meals has already been demonstrated in the case of refined grain[11]. Further, since the stomach empties continuously during the whole postprandial period, such relatively unbuffered acid strikes the duodenum, too, right from the start.

In conformity with this, I seek to show that the epidemiological distribution of peptic ulcer throughout the world accurately parallels the consumption of refined carbohydrates. Thus the disease (which cannot long remain hidden) is for all practical purposes unknown amongst the eaters of unrefined millet in Northern Nigeria and of the closely related teff in Ethiopia, and also amongst the eaters of unrefined maize, as in the Zululand Reserve of Natal. In this latter part of Africa, for example, A. Barker from the Charles Johnson Memorial Hospital, reports two cases of peptic ulcer in 25,000 consecutive in-patients. Yet in the cousins of all these Africans, the negroes in the United States, who are on a refined Westernised diet, the incidence of peptic ulcer is the same as in the whites, and in many towns in Africa, such as Nairobi, the disease is now common, following the ever-increasing consumption of refined flour and sugar. Corresponding to this latter picture in Africa is the ulcer-belt of India, but here the refined carbohydrates are mainly milled rice and manioc (tapioca). I also show that in the Japanese prisoner-of-war camps peptic ulcer was either rampant or absent, depending on whether the rice consumed was refined or unrefined, and I also draw attention to the well-documented disappearance of peptic ulcer from the German army besieged at Stalingrad, where the carbohydrates consumed became of the coarsest type.

Historically, too, the very high incidence of peptic ulcer (especially duodenal ulcer) in Westernised nations, which appeared relatively recently, around the turn of the present century, fits in well with the rise in sugar consumption, which reached the high figure of 85lb. about that time.

It will be noted that, quite apart from evolutionary considerations, none of the above evidence is compatible with stress being a primary cause of peptic ulceration, though it is shown how stress can aggravate matters by leading people to eat when they do not feel like eating. The ill-effects of this latter act, including the acid eructations it gives rise to, are also referred to by me in a later joint work[3] when discussing the aetiology of hiatus hernia.

Colonic Stasis, with Diverticular Disease and Venous Ailments

Turning now to the next site of impact of these carbohydrates, the intestines, and disregarding for the moment their absorption therefrom, the loss of fibre sustained during the refining processes has important consequences on the intestinal transit-times, which become very greatly lengthened, the stool changing from a soft narrow coil to hard, broadened masses. The reality of this stasis, especially *Colonic Stasis,* is shown by the vast consumption of aperients in Westernised countries like Great Britain, where from 15 to 30%[12, 13] or more, of all persons regularly take them. The striking aperient effect of taking raw, unprocessed bran shows how tragically the loss of this material in white flour bears on the old and the infirm, who often have neither the money nor the energy to forage for other fibre-containing foods.

I consider not only that this colonic stasis is responsible for *diverticulosis,* the forerunner of diverticulitis, which view rests partly on the absence of this condition in communities subsisting on unrefined carbohydrates, and partly on the crucial intra-colonic pressure studies by N. S. Painter[14], co-author in the later joint work[3], but also that such stasis is the dominant cause of *varicose veins* and *fermoral thrombosis*[5, 3]. For the iliac colon, and the caecum if at all distended, lie right on the external iliac veins bringing up the blood from the lower limbs, see Fig. 2. Since the colon/vein relationship is closer on the left side, especially in the recumbent position, the greater frequency of these venous disorders on the left side is explained – and without ever making the body at fault. But the main strength of the argument lies in the fact that, in races living on unrefined carbohydrates, varicose veins and femoral thrombosis are almost unknown. Thus H. Dodd[15] quotes figures supplied by A. Barker[16], from the hospital already quoted as serving a population of Africans living tribally, mainly on unrefined maize. These Africans pass a characteristic stool, soft in consistency and narrow in diameter,

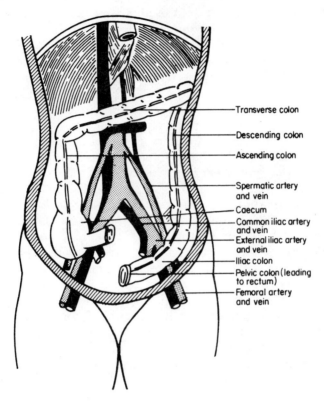

Fig. 2.—The relationship of the colon to the arteries (cross-hatched) and veins (black) at the back of the abdomen (*diagrammatic only*). (*From an original drawing by Surgeon-Commander R.J.W. Lambert, R.N.*)

twice a day, and the figures show that in 3 years, from a total of over 11,000 in-patients (including over 3,000 maternity cases) and over 100,000 out-patient attendances, there were 3 cases of varicose veins and 3 cases of femoral thrombosis. In Great Britain varicose veins form the commonest surgical complaint, some 10% of the population being afflicted with them, and post-operative and other causes of femoral thrombosis are tragically frequent and have been rapidly increasing[17].

25

A similar argument to the above readily explains the production of *haemorrhoids* and *varicocele,* the only difference being that in the former the accumulations press on veins within the bowel, running in the walls of the rectum, instead of on veins without. These two complaints are also exceedingly common in Westernised countries, but in the thousands of Africans just referred to they occurred once and three times respectively.

Finally, any racial immunity to the above venous conditions may be ruled out – *for the negroes in the United States suffer from them just as much as do the whites.*

Over-consumption: B. coli Conditions and Intestinal Toxaemia

Turning back now to the *over-consumption* that occurs with these refined carbohydrates, and still contemplating the intestinal contents, such over-consumption has a profound effect on the bacterial flora present in these contents. To take the simplest example, the stools of breast-fed infants are acid in reaction, with the B.bifidus predominant, and smell like 'bread in the oven', whereas those of infants fed on artificial mixtures, often containing heavy loads of sucrose, are alkaline in reaction, with the B.coli predominant and 'with the smell putrefying'[18,19,20]. Since the food surplus in the gut, that we are now considering, is essentially carbohydrate in nature, the resulting excess of sugar is exactly what would favour the multiplication of sugar-loving organisms like the B.coli, and in the saccharine conception the over-consumption of refined carbohydrates is regarded as the fundamental cause of *cholecystitis, appendicitis,* and primary *pyelitis* (together with the closely-related symptomless bacteriuria). And furthermore, the absorption into the bloodstream of the evil-smelling products of this bacterial decomposition is regarded as the essential cause of the intestinal toxaemia so strongly argued in the past by Ehrlich and others, of which a typical example is provided by certain skin diseases, such as some of the chronic eczemas urticarias, and perhaps by hypertension.

In connection with the above, all the epidemiological evidence shows the rarity of these B.coli infections in communities still living on unrefined carbohydrates, such as the tribal Africans already mentioned (though their cousins, the negroes in the United States, again show no such freedom). There is also the historical evidence. For example, A. Elliot[3] has shown how closely the rise in the incidence of appendicitis paralleled the rise in sugar consumption, already discussed, during a period that straddled the turn of the century.

Over-consumption: Obesity

Dealing further with the over-consumption attending refined carbohydrates, but transferring our gaze now from the intestine to the bloodstream, into which most of this surplus, as sugar, becomes absorbed, it is easy to see how closely such absorption can be related to the production of ordinary *obesity*. Indeed the saccharine conception indicates that the over-consumption of refined carbohydrate is the essential cause of this condition, which is now so common in Westernised societies that even the children are afflicted with it. There is rejected any idea that the appetite is at fault, which would mean that the body is built wrongly – and the complete absence of obesity in all wild animals, birds and fishes reinforces this rejection. There is also rejected any idea that natural desires over exercise, such as laziness, are at fault, which, again, would mean that the body is built wrongly – and a visit to any zoo similarly reinforces this rejection, for there even the interference with *desired* exercise does not seem to produce obesity as long as the food remains in its natural, unconcentrated state.

From the foregoing it is clear that salvation in obesity lies basically in taking carbohydrate foods in their natural unconcentrated state, that is, with the original fibre still in position, *and not in calculations involving calories*. At first sight it seems so logical to work out things calorifically. Thus, if the 5oz. of sugar now consumed by the average person per day in Westernised societies is contained in some 2½lb. of sugar beet, it would appear to make no difference calorifically whether one consumes the former or the latter. But, as stated earlier, this entirely ignores the all-important factors of appetite and satiety. It is easy enough to take down the 5oz. of sugar in cups of tea or as sweets, but taking down 2½lb. of sugar beet or the equivalent amount of raw fruit, such as the apples of our own temperate climate, is a very different affair. And similarly with puffy white bread, as against dense wholemeal bread. No wild animal, such as a rabbit in a whole field of grass, ever eats too much; it knows nothing about calories, but appetite and satiety, acting on unconcentrated carbohydrates, protect it infallibly. But acting on our concentrated carbohydrates, they do not protect *us*.

Over-consumption: Diabetes and Coronary Disease

Finally, as regards the above surplus of sugar entering the bloodstream, the saccharine conception indicates that this is also the essential cause of *diabetes*, through the unnatural strain imposed on the pancreas; *and because of the striking clinical association of diabetes with coronary disease*, probably the essential cause of *coronary disease*, too.

In his original paper the present writer tried to show how the difficulties in relating diabetes to carbohydrate consumption disappear if the relationship is made only with the unnatural, refined carbohydrates. Thus, during the last war the mortality from diabetes fell sharply, though total carbohydrate consumption rose – but the consumption of refined carbohydrates, through the rationing of sugar and sweets, fell sharply too.

Quite apart from the historical evidence, showing the increasing incidence of diabetes and coronary disease following in the wake of rising sugar consumption, so well presented by L. Michaels[7] in the case of coronary disease, and more accurately, in the matter of the time factor, by G. D. Campbell[21,22,23] in the case of diabetes, there is a mass of epidemiological evidence, too. This is most strikingly seen in the 250,000 Indians now living in Natal, amongst whom G.D. Campbell[23] has shown how – with most of the fats consumed being *unsaturated* – a very large increase in sugar consumption, as compared with the consumption in India, has been accompanied by a veritable explosion in the incidence of diabetes, and also of coronary disease. This evidence, together with similar evidence in Africans during their transition from a tribal to an urbanised form of existence, forms an important basis of our joint work[3]. Furthermore, the great rarity of these two diseases in tribal Africans contrasts ominously with their equal incidence in the U.S. negro and the U.S. white.

However, from the point of view of the saccharine conception, far the most important of these investigations has been the one showing the almost complete absence of diabetes in 2,000 African cane-cutters. These cutters chew the sugar cane all day long and their consumption of sugar is therefore enormous – but the sugar is nearly all in its natural dilute form. In the opinion of the present writer, this investigation is of supreme importance and presents a lasting challenge to those who do not differentiate the unnatural refined carbohydrates from the natural unrefined ones.

Saturated and Unsaturated Fats

To revert for a moment to the subject of coronary disease, and to the prevention thereof by the taking of unsaturated vegetable oils like sunflower seed oil, instead of saturated fats like butter, cream and the fat on meat, it is accepted that the present tragic frequency of this disease is a relatively new development in man's history, having mainly taken place over the last 50 years or so. Where, then, is the logic in avoiding the old-fashioned fats, to which we are evolved and which we love, and taking instead the new-fashioned oils, to which we are not evolved and which mostly we do *not* love? Thus Moses, some 3,000 years ago, stated in Deuteronomy, ch. 32, verse 14, that

Jehovah gave to his people to eat 'butter of kine, and milk of sheep with fat of lambs',* and this eating extends much further back than this – to Neanderthal man, in fact. Yet sunflower seed oil, so largely advocated these days, is derived from a plant that comes from the New World, which we and others sprung from the Old World never met until recently. Moreover, in the past most vegetable oils could seldom have been consumed as such, since it required the invention of the modern hydraulic press to enable them to be extracted from the cotton and other parent seeds. The fact that many of these oils are thus not natural foods for man lends some credibility to recent reports from the United States of increased malignant disease in those continually taking them. *Per contra* it is easy to relate coronary disease to the great rise in sugar consumption already shown. In letters to *The Lancet* setting out the above argument, the present writer also pointed out that the diseases associated with coronary disease – such as diabetes, obesity, etc. – can easily be explained by the taking of refined carbohydrates, but *not* of fats.

Note: Any surveys trying to relate coronary thrombosis to the consumption of refined carbohydrates should include *all* refined carbohydrates, since all are absorbed as monosaccharide sugars from the intestine, en route to constituting the sugar (glucose) of the blood. It would obviously be open to serious error to record sugar-consumption without referring, for example, to the maltose consumed in beer, since great numbers of people prefer 'bitters' to sweetstuffs,, yet both are equally capable of causing obesity and other diseases based on over-consumption. (*The Lancet,* 2nd January 1971, page 43.)

Renal Stone
   Is this the end of the refined-carbohydrates story? The

*Occasional biblical references to *not* eating fats concern sacrificial (burnt) offerings, since in these the fat is needed to promote the procedure adopted.

answer, unfortunately, is that it is not, for the eventual fate of these carbohydrates in the body has still to be considered. At first sight this would appear to lie in the harmless combustion of sugar into carbon dioxide and water, But a deeper look shows the sequence is not nearly as easy as that. To give the simplest example, if sugar were taken in its natural, unrefined state, it would very commonly be taken as raw fruit – and nearly all fruits, and especially the more acid ones like apples and oranges, have an *alkalising* effect on the urine. This is due to the dissipation of acid groups as carbon dioxide in the lungs, but the elimination of alkaline groups in the urine. In the consumption of refined sugar, therefore, this alkalising effect is lost and the urine becomes more acid. And this has a direct effect on the formation of *renal calculus,* since the precipitation of urates and oxalates depends more on the acidity of the urine than on almost anything else. Looking at the picture broadly, and observing the widespread effects of these refined carbohydrates on the body, as I have tried to show, it would indeed be remarkable if they did not also have an impact on the end-results of metabolism in the urine.

That the consumption of refined carbohydrates is only too likely to be the dominant cause of renal calculus is strongly supported by both historical and epidemiological evidence. As regards the former, there is – as happens in other saccharine manifestations – the big rise in the incidence in most European countries since the turn of the century, referred to in the literature as the 'stone wave'[24] of which D.A. Andersen[25] has recently produced a striking example in the case of Norway, where the condition bids fair to become 'the commonest hospital surgical abdominal disease'. And as for the epidemiological evidence, there is the well-recognised rarity of the condition in Africans living tribally on unrefined carbohydrates, but yet again the equal incidence in the U.S. negro and the U.S. white.

Part V. Line of Action Indicated

Finally, as regards the prevention and arrest of all the manifestations of the saccharine disease (but not, of course, usually the cure of damage already sustained, which may well require further measures), where does all the foregoing lead in actual practice? The answer lies in a single mode of nutrition, which embodies the careful following of natural instincts on natural foods, as I have tried to set out in the practical food guide appended to the joint work already alluded to.

In concluding this section, a plea is entered for greater simplicity in seeking the causation of the modern degenerative diseases. Is it not wise to utilise the empirical fact, first recognised by the Greeks and endorsed ever since, that simplicity holds the key to truth?

References

1. Cleave, T.L. (1956) *Journal of the Royal Naval Medical Service*, **40**, 116.
2. Cleave, T.L. (1962) *Peptic Ulcer*. Bristol: John Wright & Sons Ltd. (U.S.A.: Williams & Wilkins Co., Baltimore).
3. Cleave, T.L., Campbell, G.D. and Painter, N.S. (1969) *Diabetes, Coronary Thrombosis and the Saccharine Disease*, 2nd Edit. Bristol: John Wright & Sons Ltd. (U.S.A.: Williams & Wilkins Co., Baltimore).
4. Grundy, F. and Lewis-Faning, E. (1957) *Morbidity and Mortality in the First Year of Life*, London: Eugenics Society.
5. Cleave, T.L. (1960) *On the Causation of Varicose Veins*, Bristol: John Wright & Sons Ltd. (U.S.A.: Williams & Wilkins Co., Baltimore). Also 3 above.
6. Anter, M.A., Ohlson, M.A. and Hodges, R.E. (1964) *American Journal of Clinical Nutrition*, **14**, 169.
7. Michaels, L. (1966) *British Heart Journal*, **28**, 258.
8. MacGregor, A.B. (1964) *Annals of the Royal College of Surgeons of England*, **34**, 179.

9. Hardwick, J.L. (1960) *British Dental Journal,* **108,** No. 1, 13, 14.

10. Tovey, F.I. See 2 above, page 134.

11. Lennard-Jones, J.E., Fletcher, J. and Shaw, D.G. (1968) *Gut,* **9,** 177.

12. Morris, J.N. (1941) *The Lancet,* **1,** 51.

13. Connell, A.M., Halton, C., Irvine, G., Lennard-Jones, J.E. and Misiewicz, J.J. (1965) *British Medical Journal,* 4, 1095.

14. Painter, N.S. (1968) *American Journal of Digestive Diseases,* **13,** 468.

15. Dodd, H. (1964) *The Lancet,* **2,** 910.

16. Barker, A. (1964) *Ibid.,* **2,** 970.

17. Morrell, M.T., Truelove, S.C. and Barr, A. (1963) *British Medical Journal,* **2,** 830.

18. Naish, F.C. (1948) *Breast Feeding,* 95. London: Oxford University Press.

19. Ellis, R.W. (1960) *Diarrhoeal Diseases of Infancy,* 295. Edinburgh: E. & S. Livingstone Ltd.

20. Snyder, M.L. (1940) *Journal of Infectious Diseases,* **66,** 2.

21. Campbell, G.D. (1959). Congress Abstracts South African Medical Association, East London, 45. Published by South African Medical Association, Cape Town.

22. Campbell, G.D. (1960) *South African Medical Journal,* **34,** 332.

23. Campbell, G.D. (1963) *Ibid.,* **37,** 1195.

24. Sallinen, P. (1959) *Acta chirurgica Scandinavica,* **118,** 479.

25. Andersen, D.A. (1966) *Journal of the Oslo City Hospitals,* **16,** 101.

3. The story of a nutrient theory

Cmdr. Michael Blake

Michael Blake is a practising farmer who has written two books, 'Concentrated Incomplete Fertilisers' and 'Down to Earth, real principles for fertiliser use' which invoke rational nutrition of soils and plants. Blake believes that the health of soil, crop, animal and man are adversely affected by practices in bondage to the notorious triad NPK (nitrogen, phosphorus and potassium), and he quotes scientific authorities from whom he has drawn his evidence.

Habitat One

FOR any story which covers a century or more, perspective is a factor of importance. To understand what progress agricultural man, (and that includes his advisers), has made in shaping natural resources of his surface environment to cater for his ever-increasing demands, it is helpful that he should look at himself as a living organism in that environment: a living organism striving like all others to obtain the highest possible standard of living: but, unlike other living organisms, having at his disposal resources of energy and intellect which are not available in any other state of natural order or equilibrium.

In chemical terms the farmer has inorganic resources which have been acquired by using his organic resource of intellect. His newly acquired resources are of true energy in the form of machinery created and driven by using the Earth's reserves of fossil fuels which man mines in various forms; machinery for draining and cultivating his soils, and for manufacturing chemical substances which he applies to the surfaces of his cropping soils.

A Nutrient Theory

Four hundred years ago, in our latitude and climate, the farmer's enemy was the forest, which was indigenous to our soils and continually threatened to encroach on his agriculture. At that time the open-field farmer cropped off the fertility which natural vegetation had stored; until he exhausted that fertility, his crops failed, and weeds and shrubs took over. The 'organic' resources of that living organism (the farmer) – intuition, experience, and intellect – overcame the breakdown by enclosing land, and putting it into pasture (because it was too exhausted for arable cropping), in which form it fortuitously met the demand of a booming wool trade. Possibly the old saying 'Down corn, up horn' derived from that time.

The movement from arable to pastoral necessitated enclosure because grazing under common land tenure was, (and still is in such places as the New Forest), not a practical concern. What was unforeseen in this transition was the rejuvenation of the soil by a rest under grass, and more importantly the radical transformation of the biology of the soil from a forest to a grassland structure.

The continuous biological activity of living and dead grasses produces a grass humus which fully integrates with the mineral clay fraction of the top-soil; thus creating a characteristic crumb structure usually described as 'granular'. In such a grassland structure, air and water can percolate freely. The granules which are created by the growth and movement of the grass roots obtain porosity and absorbent capacity from the grassland humus: and this absorbent capacity is both physical and chemical: physical in its water-holding ability which helps drainage in times of flood, and reserves water for plant nutrition in times of drought: chemical in its ability to retain mineral bases of the soil for slow release for plant nutrition as the plant roots require them. This environment makes the soil ideal for bacterial as well as plant growth, and a high level of bacterial activity results in a sustained decomposition of the humus to supply all those desirable requirements. Physically, chemically, and biologically, the grassland granular soil structure has all the qualities ideal for agricultural crops.

This is quite as should be expected when it is understood that many basic crops of agriculture are derived and bred from grasses – perennials for animal grazing, and annual cereal crops for animal and human consumption.

These concepts of soil fertility have been stressed by many people, not least by Sir George Stapledon, and perhaps most perfectly and persistently by G.V. Jacks, Deputy Director of the Bureau of Soil Science, Rothamsted.

The aspect of our record which I wish to present is the story of how man has used his 'organic' resources – of skill and intellect – in applying those inorganic chemical substances for increasing the production of his agricultural soils.

Some Facts of Life

A survey of such pretensions needs to be launched from a rock-bottomed platform of chemical fact. The great fundamental is that the whole process of growth and decay of all living organisms represents, in the ultimate analysis, a continuous process of changes of chemical substance: that chemistry itself is ultimately electrical, and has therefore only two aspects – positive or negative – and because electrons are electrically charged there are only two possible states – present or absent.

Throughout chemistry all change of substance operates by gain or loss or exchange of electrons. Throughout the whole process of growth and decay such change of substance by gain or loss of electrons applies to animal bodies, plants, the microbial mass of the soil population, and the minerals of the soil. It applies also to all amendments and additions to the soil of whatever form – manures, composts, lime and the metals of bases, or concentrated salts.

Of particular relevance to this survey it should be stressed that all the electrically charged particles or groups of particles, called ions, of essential substances such as water, acids, alkalis, and salts (including fertilisers) always occur in pairs with opposite electrical charges. In soil chemistry and plant nutrition the positive ions are named cations, and the negative ions are named anions. It is both unscientific and unpractical to consider a convenient or desirable nutrient cation without at the same time considering the effects of its accompanying anion. Endless disregard of this truth is, above anything else, a principal cause of many soil fertility problems which confront agriculture today.

Fundamentally the state of the soil, fertilisers added to it, plant growth, and the production of food, are examples of electronic changes among the salts and minerals of the earth, and the gases of the atmosphere. The management of these exchanges by the farmer is the key to successful farming. The first logical step in management is to appreciate that the chemical (or electronic) transformations that are necessary to produce food depend always on having enough suitable substances in the immediate surface environment: and that thereafter in due season radiant energy from the sun will activate the chemical changes. The suitable substances are essentially sixteen elements: they comprise oxygen and carbon from the atmosphere, hydrogen from the water of soil and air, and thirteen mineral nutrients of the soil (six major and seven minor) available to plants via the soil water. These soil minerals are the substances of the soil-based metabolism of plants, which in turn provide the energy source – through assimilation as food – for animals and other living organisms including the microbial masses of the soil which carry through with decay, so that the cycle may start again and continue.

Biological chemistry or biochemistry (which is the chemistry of growth and decay) depends on two primeval facts from the earliest stages of evolution. Firstly that all life depends on water. Secondly that *oxidation* (combining with oxygen – as in animal respiration) and hydrogenation – more usually called *reduction* (combining with hydrogen – as in photosynthesis by green plants) are equal and opposite always. If any substance is reduced something else is oxidised to an equal and opposite extent.

These primeval facts are the basis of all chemical changes in the life-cycle. They lead to the concept of equivalence which is the chemical way of expressing Nature's invariable observance of balance and equilibrium. It is a general proposition of nothing for nothing, and something only for its exact chemical equivalent, whether the currency of exchange is energy or substance.

These 'facts-of-life' are not disputed. My survey sets out to examine the record of agriculture in its chemical treatment of soils and crops, and to assess the extent to which it has or has not complied with the terms upon which Nature will accept our co-operation, terms evolved through milleniums; terms which we cannot bend or twist in the least degree without loss or full payment within the concept of **equivalence**. I have not evoked the record of plant and soil nutrition by husbandry methods which follow natural order. These are influenced for good or bad by the chemical treatments imposed upon them. For instance, the re-cycling of mineral nutrients of the soil via the decay of the organic residues of crops and animals may be assisted or hindered by chemical treatments or by lack of them.

It is therefore necessary to bear always in mind that unenlightened practices with chemical fertilisers may react unfavourably, not merely against the immediate object of the practice (which is usually crop yield), but inevitably also against the efficient functioning of many kinds of living organisms, and chemical and physical processes all acting on the inorganic parent material from which our soils stem. In short, the whole nature of soil-fertility will be influenced for good or bad.

The Record

We have always relied on the mineral reserves of our soils to grow crops. For instance our 18th-century wool export trade relied on soil sulphur to supply grass with sulphate to grow the high quality grass proteins which in turn produced the high-quality wool from the back of the sheep. This was before the time of sulphur-dioxide fall-out from air pollution, and at a time when the sulphur which fell to English earth from the atmosphere did not exceed about 3lb. per acre during the growing season. Almost certainly a great deal more than this amount went into the growing of the wool. This is not a hypothetical fancy. Wool itself is 15% cysteine: cysteine is one of the essential sulphur-bearing amino-acids, and contains 27% sulphur. Extensive fall-out records conducted recently in Eire by a soils research team in conjunction with their Met. Office disclose that during the five 'growing' months April to August no more than 3 or 4 pounds of sulphur per acre falls to Irish soils. Much of South and West England may expect no more.

'Nutrient theory' was introduced in the 'fifties of last century to express nothing more than the notion that certain elements could feed plants. This 'nutrient' effect was proven by increases of yields as shown by crude experiments which usually lasted only a year or two. 'Nutrient theory' – as that sort of information was called – did not, and could not, tell anything about effects on soil or about long-term questions like maintenance of soil fertility. The 'theory' was blissfully pre-scientific.

The yield-promoting effects of nitrogen (N), phosphate (P), and potash (K) were particularly obvious and consequently became known as the 'essential' major nutrients in the embryonic nutrient theory.

Rothamsted Experimental Station made little use of NPK terminology during the lives of its founders Lawes and Gilbert in the later years of the last century. The first application of modern statistical technique evolved at Rothamsted was directed to a problem in soil bacteriology where chemicals were not involved. From about 1928, however, statistical analyses of fertiliser experiments were sent out from Rothamsted coupled with nutrient theory that had proliferated elsewhere.

D

The hollowness of nutrient theory is clearly shown by consideration in chemical terms of the ideas underlying statistical processing of treatment interactions. Nutrient theory is based on pretending that nutrients are entities capable of existing in their own right, together with the idea that fertilisers can exert effects corresponding to whatever nutrient or group of nutrients is uppermost in the experimenter's mind. N in (say) ammonium sulphate is treated as if it acts by itself. In consequence entire fertilisers that contain N are discussed and compared as if they were no more than carriers of different percentages of N.

It has, for example, been accepted that sulphate is a major nutrient. It has also been accepted that chloride in quantity promotes a growth restricting effect. In spite of this knowledge the pretence that ammonium-sulphate is effective only because of its N, and that muriate of potash (potassium chloride of which half the content is chloride) is effective only because of its potash is effectively kept up; otherwise statistical interactions such as NK between, say, ammonium-sulphate and potassium-chloride cannot be sustained.

In contrast the nutrient effects of substances which, like ammonium-phosphate, contain two of the three NPK nutrients, are recognised as difficult to study using existing statistical techniques. There is, therefore, a conflict which, obvious as it may seem, has existed for more than 40 years without an urge for reconsideration coming from any statistical centre. Until about ten years ago Rothamsted was content to denote any commercial phosphatic fertiliser not of NP type as P bare, and to conduct statistical analysis of yield responses on that basis, ignoring the undoubted nutrient effects of calcium and sulphate alike.

Why, in the face of a century of knowledge that sulphate is a nutrient, should ammonium sulphate be labelled N in order that interactions involving N can be calculated for some fertilisers, while similar treatment of ammonium phosphate ('NP') is ducked?

Chemistry is declared on all sides to be a science basic to life. In 1970 however it still appears that the use, the evaluation, the manufacture of chemical fertilisers are geared, glued, and set in maintaining the incongruities of that embryonic nutrient theory which pretends that some nutrient cations of fertilisers are entities, and that their accompanying anions such as sulphate and chloride may be of no consequence to the farmer or his soil.

Post-War Developments

Thirty years ago, NPK nutrient theory was still an acceptable compromise for the purpose of simplifying reference and practice in the use of chemical fertilisers.

Farmers were lucky then; because chemical fertilisers contained significant amounts of metallic base which (besides having actual nutrient effects) contributed towards neutralising the actions on the soil brought about by acidifying forms of nitrogen. The fertilisers also contained other mineral nutrients important for the normal metabolism of plants, animals, and the soil. In particular they supplied the important elements calcium, magnesium, and sulphur.

At the same time, lime and the old-fashioned base-sufficient fertilisers (such as basic slag, kainit, Chilean nitrates, and single superphosphate) were freely used in addition to the low-analysis compound fertilisers. Taken together such older fertilisers supplied significant amounts of all the thirteen important minerals of the soil.

Now (1970) technological progress in manufacture has succeeded in producing high-analysis (notably high-N) fertilisers which are almost pure chemicals and are also almost devoid of metallic base and trace elements and other minerals; those being collectively valuable for the well-being and growth of plants and animals and for sustained productivity of the soil. Nonetheless, such concentrated fertilisers continue to be sold, and to have large claims made for their efficacy, in the old NPK terms of nutrient theory which (however adequate NPK descriptions were many

41

years ago, as applied to the older fertilisers) quite fail to correspond to modern conditions. In fact, modern conditions of farming require a *greater* proportion (not a smaller one) of the elements in which modern concentrated fertilisers are gravely deficient.

Today, intensive and extractive cropping of plants and its corresponding intensity of livestock output is setting up bigger demands upon the so-called 'uneconomic' mineral nutrients (including trace elements) from the soil. This word 'uneconomic' means, in this connection, those soil-saving and nutrient elements which manufacturers of modern concentrated fertilisers find it inconvenient or impossible to supply in their goods – though they were supplied in fair proportion in the older fertilisers which it is now convenient or fashionable to decry. However, sales of fertilisers as a whole indicate that less lime and old-fashioned fertilisers are in fact being used – and this is happening at a time when the need for education about the importance of elements which they supply has become greater than ever. Such words as 'economic' thus suggest that instead of giving detailed attention to the real needs of good farming, we have become the mouthpieces of advertising copy-writers schooled in types of industrial economics which are grossly inadequate when applied to biological aspects of soil-fertility. Consequently a great deal of injudicious advice continues to be reiterated by some merchants and distributors, and by agricultural journalists and advisers

Although it is still possible to engage in arable or mixed farming by trusting to luck that the soil will provide, for a time, those safeguards which NPK nutrient theory says nothing about, and modern concentrated N and NPK fertilisers do not cater for, the stock of sustaining fertility elements must inevitably be depleted. Such philosophy is out-dated. It may still satisfy some farmers for a few seasons yet on the lighter soils, and those on well stocked clay soils for a generation perhaps. To continue to draw on soil capital in this manner is bad business and bad economics.

At this juncture in farming, particular care is necessary in all education and reference to the use of fertilisers. Among other things, it should be forcefully brought to the notice of farmers that intensive and persistent use of fertilisers creates a greatly increased requirement for the necessary lime and other elements of which these fertilisers are supplying less and less.

Unfortunately, at this critical time, economics of fertilisers manufacture are the economics of industry. It is the technology of synthesising concentrated salts, and eliminating the handling of bulky substances. In short, a move under intense competition, *away from* the evolved requirements of the soil, plants, and animals. This is understandable and probably inevitable, but there are those in commercial agriculture under these pressures, (and often under a façade of science) who seem not to dare to warn farmers of the complementary work and cost of sustaining fertility with bulky earthy substances when concentrated fertiliser salts are used intensively: and by so failing, tend to guide practice back to a much earlier century by relying on the capital of the soil for ten or more essential elements.

1850 was the starting time of NPK theory. Since then, a great deal has come to notice about soil-chemistry such as the effects of various plant nutrients and fertiliser programmes and cropping systems on soil, and about other matters which go further than merely supplying 'nutrients'. When taken together these new indications of science (those more recent than 'nutrient' theory, that is) are valuable pointers towards the right conduct of farming as a whole. But none of what can now be seen to be indispensable information ever came into the early ideas about feeding plants: nor is it possible for those symbols NPK to indicate anything except the mere percentages of those nutrients in fertilisers. In short, by relying on NPK, any knowledge beyond the percentages of those three ingredients is lost; and farmers are deprived of much possible benefit. If the nutrients have an effect besides the benefit they are supposed to have for crops, the effect is not disclosed. It follows that if any fertiliser has effects which an advertiser does not wish farmers to know about (for example a large content of chloride), the best thing (from the selling point of view) that the advertiser can do is to lean heavily on statements about its N, P, and K and to hope that farmers will then be trusting enough to be satisfied and will not ask questions which might be awkward from the point of view of sales.

For instance, it became known as long ago as 1856, and from analyses of soil receiving nothing but organic manures, that nitrogen in even low-analysis fertilisers could rob the soil of valuable bases and thus make the farmland more acid, whenever a fertiliser itself did not contain a proper amount of mineral base. Further experiments have proved that this acidifying effect of base-poor fertilisers depends upon a fundamental and inescapable truth. Acids are invariably formed in soils, so that the soil is impoverished by use of fertilisers, *unless* enough base to neutralise all the possible acidity is *either* present in the fertilisers (whatever their kind or origin) *or* is added as an extra (conventionally by liming only). If the soil is chalky, the same base-stealing effect still happens, although it may be hidden for a while. The fertility-sustaining elements which then leach out are calcium, magnesium, sodium, and potassium; and in addition some important trace elements – copper in particular.

The high calcium content of chalk soils is necessarily accompanied by a proportionately lower content of three other principal soil minerals (or bases), magnesium, potassium, and sodium. Losses of exchangeable calcium over chalk soils from acid formation will always predominate; but, because of the large reserves of calcium, these losses are not so important as the losses of magnesium, potassium, and sodium, which are 'naturally' in chronic short supply. Since conventional doctrine (of lime only for replenishment of soil bases) declares liming to be unnecessary for calcareous soils, no further consideration appears to be given to replenishment of those other bases in chronic short supply:

excepting potash which happens to be 'included' in nutrient theory.

For many chalk-land farmers these reminders come especially near home, since their soils often consist of a thin layer of permeable soil lying on a bed of chalk which does almost nothing to protect the cropped layer from washing-out of the scarce bases, magnesium, potassium and sodium, whenever base-poor (but nitrogen-rich) manures are supplied by the farmer to his crops. In view of the sales pressure on fertilisers carrying high percentages of nitrogen but practically no base of any kind, it is no wonder that a dramatic falling-away of corn crops has quickly made itself evident on many soils over chalk.

In spite of all the knowledge that science has brought forward about soils and fertilisers, and in spite of the length of time much of it has been known, very little of this useful knowledge has lately been allowed to reach farmers by being put honestly before them.

The Farmer's Problem

It is important that every farmer should have the opportunity to understand some results that flow from adherence to an out-dated and unhelpful NPK theory of fertilising. The results penetrate the whole of farming by being potentially bad for soil, crops, and animals, and consequently for the farmer's pocket.

It is perhaps not of the first importance whether belief in NPK as a sufficient description of fertilisers is held by the farmer himself as a carry-over from old and different times; but it matters very much when he is appealed to on such a doubtful basis as NPK in advertisements and other propaganda which claim to inform him of science-based developments in fertilising, and when the farmer has no means of detecting whether the *implications* of the advertised figures are in any way worthy of trust. Farmers should be able to have complete confidence that the fertilisers they buy will not in either the long or the short run be harmful to their farm or their pockets.

If farmers are not to be the victims, the onus for buying wisely should not be left with them – as it, unfortunately, now is. In selling and buying fertilisers the bad old principle of *caveat emptor* (let the buyer beware) continues – about many matters which intimately concern the farmer – unchecked. Some good could be done by extending farm education about the properties of fertilisers: and not only about what they contain but about what the absence of certain constituents could mean all round the farm; but that alone would not suffice, and farmers cannot be expected to be chemists. However, farmers have every right to expect not to have advantage taken of them because they do not have a wide-ranging scientific knowledge.

It would be much fairer – and far more helpful to every farmer – if all manufacturers supplied, with every purchase, a full description of what the goods consist of and what the probable outcome would be for the soil if it is applied to the land. (Acidifying, or not requiring lime, for example). That represents no new principle; it has been followed in retailing many kinds of merchandise where consumers have to be protected. A system of full labelling does not mean anything more than that the manufacturers should share with their customers the up-to-date and fully scientific knowledge the manufacturers already possess – instead of trying to pull wool over farmers' eyes by the reiterated pretence that NPK alone can give a useful description.

The present regrettable tendency is of recent origin; it is essentially no older than the modern 'concentrated' fertilisers, and has in effect grown up with them and has accompanied the development of such concentrated materials unhindered by 'official' caution. It is nonetheless an attempt to blind farmers with last century's 'science' by quoting only figures for N, P, and K – which, in any case, no longer hold the meanings that could reasonably be attached to them last century and up to World War II (before concentrated fertilisers were made).

Amid our modern civilisation, it is a stunning fact – not yet brought home to the majority of farmers and growers – that the legal provisions about fertilisers that were drawn up to protect against a widespread evil of adulteration last century (and have effectively given the protection) are now employed to uphold out-dated chemical ideas that encourage the continuance of much agronomically-dubious farming practice in totally different circumstances; with the effect, almost, of offering up land and the farming community as a sacrifice to the industrial economics of fertiliser manufacture. The, perhaps, unconscious manner in which this happens is more insidious and subtle than the earlier adulteration because it appeals to a fetish of 'purity', and proceeds without any sign of alertness or check by independent Governmental or Government-supported agencies supposedly teaching and acting on behalf of farmers.

Farmers' Costs

A further serious weakness of NPK or nutrient theory in its application to current farming practice is that the almost pure ingredients of modern fertilisers (in forms not disclosed by the sellers) are sold, bought, considered, and used for production of the annual crop; it being the annual crop and the farmer's resulting net annual income which mainly comprise the realm wherein the bargaining between farmer and Government takes place, and whereby farmers' prices are established.

After harvest (when the annual crops have been removed) additional operations involving the purchase and distribution of further 'nitrogen' (also in forms possibly not known to the farmer), and also lime and other fertility-sustaining materials, are generally necessary if white straw residues are to be successfully incorporated in the soil by being broken down into a state which (in six months' time) will assist the growth of the next year's crop, and not actually hinder it.

These aspects of farmers' budgeting involve two considerations which are of great importance to the corn farmer (at least), but about which nutrient theory is silent. It is silent for the good reason that nutrient theory (which the legally-based propaganda for concentrated fertilisers still invites us to believe in as the last word about fertilising) evolved long before either pH and the equally important subject of carbon-nitrogen ratio in soil were thought of; so a description in terms of no more than NPK cannot tell anything useful at all about some important aspects of the fertiliser to which it is attached.

In brief, the farmer becomes involved in extra work and costs to maintain not only soil reaction or acidity at a favourable level but also to make sure that the ratio of carbon and nitrogen in the soil is right. These two things go together; for the decomposition of stubble, a ley, or whatever is ploughed under, contributes essentially to the maintenance of the soil organic content and the formation of humus: and that decomposition, contributing positively to soil structure, cannot proceed satisfactorily and rapidly enough if the soil is deficient in lime – as it well may be if the farmer gives nothing but concentrated fertilisers to the main crop, or to grass about to be ploughed up.

Is the 'balance sheet' of soil fertility considered at all during the annual bargaining for farmers' prices? A farmer's 'net annual income' takes into account all the savings in costs (including labour and streamlining his system) that he makes under great economic pressure. It is this realm – of immediate or year-to-year prices and costs – which seems to preside over the table around which farmers' prices are argued; and nothing much is said about deterioration or improvement of the soil which is the farm capital in land.

It is more than debatable that such a system of taking short aims has disguised some broad declines and deficits in the annual 'balance-sheets' of fertility. It is probably these which are subtly and, as it were, invisibly (subclinically) manifested in some states of animal health;

though such states are only too visible when they require veterinary attention. In animal husbandry the prevailing jungle of corrective measures (veterinary intervention and dietetic supplements) provides clear evidence that many fertiliser practices have been pressured into disregard of numerous essential requirements of herbage, animals, and soil. This has been done under the pretence that in home-produced fodder only the quantity of dry matter and its crude protein are 'economic' considerations; but since the fodder will have been produced on land which may have received little more than the NPK supplied in the latest way by modern fertilisers, it looks as if to that extent we are still prisoners of NPK theory as vouchsafed by the fertiliser manufacturers – there being, apparently, nobody to tell the farmer about the animal requirements that could be completely supplied by a rational policy about fertilising.

The cost of inorganic supplementary feeding with substances which could more effectively be supplied as organic compounds in herbage and which were once to a large extent supplied by fertilisers (to be cycled to livestock by that route), is overlooked on short-term views. Ironically, there is a tendency to take such unnecessary extra outlays as part of the 'progressiveness' of farming to-day! The potential run-down of the soil itself is equally overlooked.

The Manufacturer's Problem

In the old days compound fertilisers were made by simply mixing fertilisers together, as for example sulphate of ammonia, superphosphate and muriate of potash, and there is no scientific difficulty in specifying the composition of the mixture. But many present-day compounds are made by dissolving an ammonium phosphate and muriate of potash in molten ammonium nitrate, and though it is quite easy to say what went into the mix, it is very difficult to say what actual chemical compounds are present in the mix, when it is sold to the farmer, because of changes that may take place in the molten mix. The problem becomes still more difficult with compounds of uncertain composition, such as nitro-phosphate fertilisers.

Coming down to detail, it is essential that a farmer should know in what form his nitrogen is present, whether as ammonium, nitrate, or urea, and particularly when he is dealing with ammonium sulphate and ammonium nitrate or urea fertiliser (all acid-forming). If, in the future, slow-acting nitrogen fertilisers, such as oxamide or substituted ureas come on to the British market, it will also be important to declare what proportion of the nitrogen is present in such uncompensated forms.

The ammonium in ammonium sulphate, ammonium nitrate or an ammonium phosphate, and an ammonium magnesium phosphate, may all behave differently in a soil; a base rich sodium nitrate will behave differently again, and urea still differently. So it is essential that the farmer should know more or less what the principal nitrogen compounds in the fertiliser are. The actions of these compounds are probably not greatly affected by the presence of other PK materials in the fertiliser. For potassium the other part of the potassium salt can be very important, and in particular it is important to know if it is chloride, sulphate, nitrate or polyphosphate. Up to the present it has always been present as chloride unless the manufacturer has definitely said it was as sulphate (which is more expensive); but should the nitrate or the metaphosphate become popular – and they are being manufactured commercially on a small scale in other countries – it would become important to know the form of the potassium, and a statement of the potassium salt added to the mixed fertiliser would give the information the farmer wanted.

The problem of phosphate is much more difficult, because as soon as one has left the simple single or triple superphosphates and ammonium ortho-phosphates (the ammonium phosphate fertilisers of present-day commerce in Great Britain) the chemical form of phosphate, and consequently its manurial value under different soil and climatic conditions, become much less precise and definite.

Examples of the problem arise in trying to specify the exact form of the phosphate in nitro-phosphates – which are phosphates made by treating rock phosphate with nitric or hydrochloric acid instead of sulphuric acid. These are not sold in Great Britain yet, though they are in some other countries; but if the price of sulphuric acid continues to rise could become very attractive financially (for the manufacturers) in many parts of this country if some minor manufacturing problems are overcome. Again, it is still not possible to specify the exact chemical composition of a polyphosphate or the so-called metaphosphates, nor yet are methods available for assessing their fertiliser value on different soils, but it is quite possible that methods for assessing their manurial value will be developed long before methods for assessing their exact chemical composition. Thus the mere information that a fertiliser contains say 15% of potassium metaphosphate would not tell the farmer much about the manurial value of the metaphosphate, though it is quite possible that a guarantee of the per cent of phosphate soluble in a certain solution might be of great value.

This discussion on fertiliser chemistry indicates that it is possible in the future that the chemistry of our fertilisers may become much more complicated and it may become scientifically increasingly difficult to say exactly what chemical products are present in the fertiliser. It may therefore remain more important to have guarantees of solubilities than of chemical composition. Any change in legislation on fertiliser composition should take account of possible future developments in fertiliser technology and not stifle new developments. It can already be argued that our present legislation, demanding the specification of water soluble and total phosphate only and therefore making dicalcium phosphate financially unattractive to the farmer, is costing the country several millions of pounds a year unnecessarily; and one would not want to introduce new legislation that would hinder the development of cheaper fertilisers.

The Industrial Economics of Fertiliser Manufacture versus the Evolved Requirements of Soils, Plants and Animals (M versus SPA)

What the manufacturers claim about the actual composition and chemistry of present and future fertilisers emphasises the difficulties of deciding, by analysis or otherwise, what is actually contained in the current 'high-analysis' fertilisers or in the coming nitro-phosphates. It illustrates the manufacturers' problems – rather than the practical and productive problems of farmers.

It has clearly become more difficult to state what are the actual compounds (chemical compounds or substances, that is) than it was in the days when mixed fertilisers other than kainit (sold as mined) were simple mixtures (each ingredient having a knowable, if not always declared, composition). Nor should the advance of 'science' (= fertiliser technology) impose on the farmer-user the burden of becoming familiar with new technicalities such as the difference, if any, between ortho- and meta-phosphate.

This discussion on fertiliser chemistry is concerned with the question of saying exactly what chemical *products* are present. The farmer is surely concerned less with analytical niceties or chemical denominations than with what the effects will be on his soil, crops, and livestock. About that all-important matter, the manufacturers are silent. Another way of putting this cardinal objection is to say that their approach is still, (after 120 years), taken up with *plant-nutrient* effects only.

Since soil and crops are mainly vehicles for nutrition of animals (the crops themselves may show shortages of some nutrient elements or may show lack of normal balance in soil condition) it might be extraordinary to let the farm animals pass without a fair crack of the whip – that is, if it were not so usual to do so! On the nutrient front there seems to be no effective mention of sulphate which it is indispensable to supply to plants for the well-being of animals. Sulphate, like calcium, is one of those ingredients or nutrients which are apparently awkward to supply in modern high-analysis fertilisers. (There is a new process whereby ammonium sulphate is added to a high-analysis mix; but that is for some purely mechanical or conditioning purpose like assisting granulation).

It is a little alarming to say the least, that all these modern fertilisers – and, presumably, those to which the manufacturers look forward as yet to come – are introduced on the nation-wide commercial scale without regard to anything except their content of N, P, and K; and without serious trial of any kind. Nor does old-fashioned knowledge (such as that about nitrification) give valid support to NPK-based allegations about the agronomic sufficiency of such fertilisers. The outstanding example of all that is liquid ammonia. A recent example of the sort of instruction among farmers which experience shows is needed is the warning by R.W. Pearson and B.D. Doss, of Alabama: 'Acid subsoils stop cotton roots, in 'Progressive Farmer' based on *Agron. J.*, Vol. 39, Sept-Oct. 1967, 453-456.

The exact wording of the warning is:

> 'Subsoil acidity is a common problem throughout the region (of the South-eastern United States), and is being intensified by use of high rates of acid-forming fertilisers without a balanced liming program.'

> And (it goes on): 'Strongly acid subsoils are a serious problem because there is no practical means of properly mixing lime with subsoil. Surface-applied limestone generally moves downward in soil at a very slow rate so that it may take many years to reduce subsoil acidity in this way.'

In other words: Subsoil acidity (not necessarily of very high order: say pH 5.0 about) may take a long time to show itself after use of high rates of high-N fertilisers; but once it declares itself (by pH soil-testing or poor growth or rooting of crops) it will be difficult and expensive to correct (by something like subsoil ploughing and heavy liming (both)).

Although the requirement for better instruction about liming and *other* methods of base replenishment has increased, official British interest in it seems to have declined; at least there seems to have been little to match the increasing use of liquid ammonia. This may be exemplified by the liming record of my own county, Hampshire.

In the single county of Hampshire, during the last ten years the amount of lime of all sorts applied by farmers has fallen more than 50% from 126,000 tons in 1959 to 56,000 tons in 1968: in the same period the number of acres limed has fallen even more seriously from about 50,000 to less than 20,000.

What now happens (with nitrogenous fertilisers especially) is that the advertisers can quite legally pull wool over farmers' eyes by relying on the chemistry of the middle of last century. Surely, no other industry besides farming is having to run on technological principles legally supported by 'progressive' ideas of a hundred years ago – and with no injection of any more recent knowledge: all of which new knowledge can be flouted with impunity?

Nobody will dispute that all fertilisers and fertilising without exception depend absolutely on ionisation (since plants cannot take up any nutrient not ionised). To this simple but fundamental knowledge – which is in no way made use of by NPK ideas – there has to be added some qualitative knowledge, such as the essentiality of certain sulphur compounds obtained by animals from plants; and the inescapable acid-forming effects of nitrification.

Hence the whole story of fertilising – from factory to soil and animals – could be stated from rock-bottom first principles; yet no official attempt has been made to make a push away from NPK and that sort of thing, including the apologetics put forward about analytical impossibilities and awkwardnesses for manufacturers.

Farmers have suffered a great deal from official inattention even to current practice. So, commercial continuous cereal-growing took the research stations unawares; so did 'high-analysis' fertilisers take the advisory centres (at least in England) unawares about the matters of liming and magnesium sodium and sulphur deficiencies. So, I suspect will nitro-phosphates find official centres unprepared to take up new questions of sulphur-deficiency (unless the use of the present almost sulphur-free concentrated fertilisers brings it to notice before nitro-phosphates become common).

Amend the Act

In 1968, with assistance from Dr. Hugh Nicol, F.R.I.C., F.R.S.E., (a specialist in ionic aspects of soil chemistry nutrition), I put forward proposals for amending the laws of description under the Fertiliser Act, 1926. These proposals were adopted as official policy by the National Farmers Union. As a first step the proposals called for a legal requirement for a declaration of .the content of calcium, magnesium, sodium, sulphate, and chloride in addition to NPK: including NIL declarations. Also some indication of the neutralisation requirement of the contents of the whole bag: and that the form of nitrogen should also be declared.

The proposals were intended as positive steps towards improving the present state which allows truth and fable about fertilisers and their effects over the whole farm to struggle for the comprehension of technical matters by farmers. For this fight – very unequal as it must be – there are no appropriate rules governing manufacturers; nor is there any intervention by a referee. Indeed no such referee exists: the official advisory services and research stations do not seem to take any positive action towards watching that farmers are not knocked down by a foul, although the rule-book should be well known to scientists. Even less, in the settlement of farmers' prices, is account taken of soil factors which are important for production and are made or marred by the fertilisers used or not used.

Last century's nutrient theory is a wretched foundation for building a policy of progressive farming.

The *effects* of fertilisers proceed from their actual composition. There should be no mercy for attempts to fob off any farmer with supposition and guesswork about matters so vitally important as the composition and total effects of the fertilisers he uses. The present law is inadequate for this protective purpose; indeed, it leaves the door wide open to declaring only the sort of information which is now of little value to the practising farmer and may, at best, mislead.

The information which should be accessible to all farmers would lay particular emphasis on acidifying effects. Those effects are – unless the farmer takes particular care to neutralise them in special operations separate from buying and using the fertilisers – practically inescapably associated with the modern high-N fertilisers, as well as with some others. It is therefore desirable that the extra work and costs associated with these fertilisers should be plainly pointed out (instead of being hidden or grotesquely turned into some advantage of 'saving labour' by buying concentrated fertilisers). The acidifying (lime-demanding) and the opposite (lime-sparing) effects of fertilisers should be stated under the head of 'neutralising factor'. That would not be difficult for any farmer to understand, and presents no difficulty for a manufacturer to specify along with other information needed by the farmer.

If the publishing of information were carried no further than what was typically outlined in the proposals put forward, it would certainly lead to a much better understanding firstly by farmers and secondly by their advisers about what is being done by using fertilisers. Farmers would then have information far beyond what is at present obscurely afforded by statements of N, P, and K percentages; for one thing, farmers could tell whether their chosen fertilising programme would be likely to meet the needs of their soil and their livestock. It can hardly be too often emphasised that the present system of declaring only percentages of the three elements, N. P and K is based on ancient views of fertilisers as 'nutrients' for plants alone;

by adhering to that antiquated system the needs of livestock and of the soil itself are not considered at all.

The bare knowledge of the existence of the ingredients of fertilisers (and, rather importantly, of the absence of crucial ingredients therefrom) should lead to proper concern about the real effects of those fertilisers all round the farm.

Time to Get Cracking

Two years have passed since my 1968 proposals were accepted by the National Farmers Union as official policy. At present, however, prospects of progress in these directions are not encouraging. The administration of the 1926 Fertiliser Act, the laws for registration of fertilisers, and the operation of the Fertiliser Subsidy are integral features of fertiliser policies and practices. Because so many fertiliser practices stem from a constricted and outdated NPK nutrient theory, it can scarcely be hoped that the functioning of the Act and the payment of subsidies will contribute to progress. For instance, merely providing a subsidy for conventional liming is no substitute for explaining why calcium (both from lime and other materials such as basic slag), and important bases and nutrients other than NPK are today required all along the line in increasing amounts.

The whole commercial scene seems to have become fossilised in the method of statistical analysis of most aspects of fertiliser trials, manufacture, sales and usage. The effort necessary to crack this inertia seems to be hampered by discussion of items under trades descriptions clauses which appears to take up too much of the time of the Fertiliser Act Standing Committee.

The terms of reference of the Fertiliser Act Advisory Committee are to advise the Minister on the operation of the Fertiliser Act, 1926, and of changes necessary to bring the schedules of the Act into line with current practice. So long as current practice is geared to outdated theory how may any Advisory Committee be expected to give a lead? Again if the principal business of the Committee is petty agenda should scientists from remote research institutes be expected to give up valuable time to travel to Westminster to attend the meetings?

By all logic and science should not the greater part of fertiliser practice, and with it the greater part of fertiliser subsidies relate primarily to long-term fertility of the soil? In other words the **balance sheet** of soil fertility: and thereafter the lesser part of fertiliser practice be directed to regulating the annual crop? That is, a case for including the use and effects of only nitrogen, active phosphate, and from now on sulphur (in proportion) in the annual profit or loss account. At present the whole fertiliser subsidy is included in the annual Price Review Award (the profit or loss account), and this includes important sustaining fertility elements (e.g. calcium) which may take a year or two to become satisfactorily fixed in the soil.

The Fertiliser Act Advisory Committee is the ideal body to give a lead in separating the long and the short-term aspects of fertiliser practice by advising the Minister to do just this. Such a lead would go a long way to eliminating that obsession with only the plant-nutrient effects of fertilisers; an obsession which, as I pointed out at the beginning of this chapter, persistently disregards fundamental chemical truths. The persistence of our out-dated nutrient theory was illustrated in April 1970 when a member of the House of Commons asked the Parliamentary Secretary to the Minister of Agriculture by what amount he estimated the use of fertilisers would decline that year. In reply the Parliamentary Secretary estimated that in the year ending May 1970 the consumption of fertilisers would increase by about 35,000 'nutrient' tons – an increase of about 2%. The answer, of course, referred only to the NPK content of mostly concentrated fertilisers.

The answer was, of course, political. It did not take into account those mineral nutrients not considered 'economic' (see p. 42): that is to say calcium, magnesium and sulphur

58

particularly. It did not take into account the heavy losses of soil minerals which inevitably accompany the use of the modern concentrated high-nitrogen fertilisers. Thus it did not mention that, for certain, not less than half the 'nutrient' N tonnage was wasted and lost by leaching out; or that in the process every ton of 'nutrient' N that was lost took away with it between three and four tons of important mineral bases from our agricultural soils. It was silent about the fact that for every 'nutrient' ton of the most usual form of K (potassium) an equal tonnage of chloride was also applied; and that virtually all the chloride leached out of the soil rapidly taking with it also an equal tonnage of mineral base. These are chemical truths which are not accounted; remaining in that classification of 'persistent disregard'.*

An enlightened answer might have been politically a non-point or minus score, but the official answer at least provides an example of the misleading sorts of information with which farmers are bombarded from all sides. Thus such a down-to-earth matter as the fertility of our agricultural soils has become a political plaything. The twist of that story is perhaps in the tail. The P.S. was a farmer. Perhaps he, too, did not understand, and had become a victim of the NPK doctrine poured out in sales propaganda which continues to pass without comment from his own official agricultural advisers.

Habitat Two

Habitat One told how man's 'organic' resources of mind achieved a radical change of the biology of our soils from forest to that grassland structure which is so adaptable to agricultural crops. The technical part of my story disclosed some long-term effects which uninformed use of chemical substances may have on the mineral nutrients of the soil which are stored in that granular aggregate.

Habitat Two takes a look at a different soil structure

*For a full account of how these losses occur see Reference 1.

which is practically worthless for agriculture. In the language of soil science, or pedology, it is a podzol. It is a forest structure which is fertile for coniferous trees, and for some surface plants such as heath which can thrive on very poor soils.

In a coniferous forest the flora produces an acid humus which does not become integrated with the mineral clay fraction of the top-soil, (as happens with grassland humus), but forms a peaty layer above it. Surface water draining through the layer of peaty humus dissolves humic acids, which at once combine with the minerals of the soil beneath, carry away almost everything useful for plant growth, and leave a layer of near sterile white or silver sand soil. Lower down, the humic acids fall out of solution, depositing the minerals with which they combined in a layer which is compact, dark brown in colour, and richer in 'borrowed' nutrients. In such a way the forest humus makes a barren topsoil in which competitors cannot thrive, and accumulates a nutrient supply in the subsoil where the tree roots may obtain it.

If the reader notes any similarity between those processes of natural equilibrium (in which the conifer has secured its habitat by creating a barren top-soil), and some long-term effects of the unenlightened use of modern concentrated nitrogen fertilisers, or fertilisers containing large amounts of chloride, which also result in the carrying away of the mineral nutrient reserves of our agricultural top-soils – then I feel obliged to say that the parallel is wholly intentional.

I am not setting out to say that we are rapidly turning our lighter cropping soils into Surrey heathland: or that contemporary practice is deliberately setting out to destroy, in the interest of short-term gain, what has been built up by traditional conservative farming. It is, however, indisputable that through inadequate information about the contents of modern fertilisers, and through lack of advice, and through misleading advice about how those contents will injure their soils in the long-term, many farmers are being pressured into promoting just those sorts of total effects which, if carried far enough, would lead to such undesirable consequences. For instance, loss of that granular structure which is the biological essence of fertility is already widespread: and has been accompanied by an unprecedented erosion of the mineral nutrients of cropping layers of the soil: which together add up to declining soil fertility.

Indeed it is the differential loss of soil minerals by such routes that upsets Nature's normal practice of equilibrium and balance among the mineral elements; it being the resulting imbalance (unfavourable to any kind of agriculture) which is the principal contributor to those many states of metabolic disorders in plants, and in the animals which consume them: including impaired cellular structure (which means 'disease') in both.

In chemical terms these failures may be classified as the misuse of inorganic resources of chemical substance and energy by man the living organism. As to the future: man's organic resources of mind need to be directed towards creating a biological surface environment for agriculture based on improved and sustained levels of fertility. This means discarding all those short-term economics of annual budgeting which are dominated by a traditional and unseeing desire for the cheapest food from any source at any moment – produced under any conditions, or dumped or subsidised by a foreign exporter: and to give far more attention to a long-term 'balance-sheet of soil fertility' concept worked out soundly within those laws of chemical equivalence. It follows inevitably that a sound and true foundation for an agriculture controlled by Government, (as our is), will require for farm products prices which take into account the full and proper costs of sustaining that balance sheet of soil fertility in good heart.

References

1. Blake, M., *Down-to-earth*. Crosby Lockwood, London, 1970.

2. Jacks, G.V., Humus and the farmer, *Journal of the Royal Society of Arts,* 1941, Vol. 89 (No. 4582), pp. 229-239: a judicious account of forest and farm, debating the point that 'a great difference between the activities of plants and men in creating soils fit for their respective communities is that the former are co-ordinated . . . whereas the latter are, in the present stage of agricultural evolution, largely unco-ordinated.'

4. Utilisation: an essential element in nutrition

Innes H. Pearse, M.D.

Dr. Pearse is the Medical Director of the Pioneer Health Centre which she founded with her late husband, Dr. Scott Williamson. They are the joint authors of 'Science, Synthesis and Sanity' which explains the theory on which the famous Peckham Experiment was based.

DESPITE the vast and rapidly accumulating information deriving from detailed analyses of food constituents and of their consumption in closely controlled conditions, our knowledge of the utilisation of nutrients in the changing circumstances of living is still inadequate.

In view of this as yet imperfect understanding of the subject, let us set aside for the moment the stock of itemised analyses, so invaluable in disclosing the central factors in disease, and collect together some evidence to be drawn from more general surveys of the performance of the living organism – human or animal – in its environment.

The Observations of Weston Price

First let us look at man in his natural environment uninfluenced by modern civilisation. We cannot do better than begin with the survey made by Weston A. Price published in U.S.A. in 1945 under the title of *Nutrition and Physical Degeneration,* with a Foreword by Ernest Albert Hooton, Professor of Anthropology, Harvard University.[1]

Weston Price, a dentist of some eminence, was disturbed by the degenerative features of patients so repeatedly observed in his own practice. He determined to seek out, before it was too late, pockets where there might still be found people living in primitive conditions untouched by Western civilisation. For some years he devoted the long vacation to visiting no less than 14 different groups of peoples ranging from Alaska to Africa, remote Swiss valleys to Polynesia, Australian aborigines to people living in the high bare mountains of Peru, comparing where possible those in isolated situations with others of the same race already touched by modern civilisation. His evidence is the more impressive being copiously illustrated by photographs showing a quite startling comparison between the individuals in the two categories.

Everywhere the same findings were observed. Perfect jaws, perfect dentition, good skeletal structure among the primitive peoples; dental decay, deformities of jaws and bony facial formation, of the skull and often deformities of general skeletal development among those who had taken to imported food. Further evidence showed that, where, for instance, T.B. had been practically unknown, within 5 years of the consumption of the food of modern civilisation there was 15% – 20% of T.B. among the people. The weight of evidence from peoples in such very different climes and living circumstances is arresting.

Similar findings to these were given to me in 1949 by the Medical Officer of Health of Reykjavik. When I inquired about the children's teeth in his city, he answered '. . . the same as yours'. He added that before leaving on a world tour, he had spent the six previous months reviewing all the skulls in the Museum in Reykjavik, with the Professor of Anatomy. 'Until 60 years ago there was no skull without a full and perfect dentition – apart from the accidental loss of a tooth or two due to injury. Since that date there is barely one perfect jaw with all the teeth intact'. Modern transport could not have reached Iceland until about 70 years before his examination of the skulls. The same story again but from a different locality and source.

What is interesting in Weston Price's findings is the very

different nature of food intake in the widely diverse groups he visited. There is no one food that could be taken to sustain health; no need to eat 'an apple a day' or drink a pint of milk as is vulgarly supposed. In the remote Yukon area where white men die of scurvy, the indigenous peoples have avoided it by drinking infusions of the terminal shoots of spruce. Others in the far North, on the rare occasion of killing a moose in the long winter, immediately extract the adrenal glands and cutting them up share out raw slices to each member of the family. We now know the adrenals have an exceptionally high vitamin C content. Where butter and oils are unobtainable, the eyes and heads of (river) fish have kept the isolated inhabitants free from the blindness due to vitamin A deficiency.

The variety of diets recorded is immense – Australian aborigines eating only small animals, insects and wild plants; the Hebrideans, sea foods and oatmeal with but few summer vegetables; in the high Swiss valley, milk, milk products, rye bread and scanty vegetables; in Africa, blood, milk, grain and green vegetables. All these different diets have sustained robust, healthy structure of bone from generation to generation.

In Weston Price's investigation, so far flung in its world-wide scope, each locality – though different – yielded the same evidence of degeneration of structure on the arrival of modern foods. There is no evidence of any single food substance, i.e. no substance consistently recognised as dangerous, that could be held responsible for findings everywhere so similar. But all had received refined flour, refined sugar and tinned foods. It is on these that suspicion falls. We may safely take the total consumption of those substances in each case as being *quantitatively* in excess of the average amount of food (in terms of calories) that for generations had previously been available for each of the groups examined. The cause of the degeneracy was therefore unlikely to have been due to any quantitative shortage of food. But in those days of transport over long distances by sea, the food inevitably must have been sterilised by one method or another. For instance, in the preservation and storage of flour for commercial purposes, it is necessary to eradicate the germ, removing with it the valuable germ oil and husk[2] both of which are now known to have important properties for the maintenance of health. Recently, to allow the germ to be retained during milling, a technical convenience – sterilisation of the wholemeal – after the grinding has been adopted. In either case the flour is 'dead' and so suffers the disadvantages of the substitute foods that had become available to the primitive peoples observed by Weston Price.

Weston Price's surveys cover the ecological conditions necessary for enquiry into the utilisation of food capable of sustaining human health. Whereas the aetiology of disease may be disclosed by the presentation, or withdrawal, of single items of the diet exhibited 'pure', or sterilised, it is unlikely that the essential factors in the maintenance and cultivation of health will be disclosed by such methods.

The Pottenger Experiment

In view of the inference that freshness of food had some bearing on the maintenance of the structure and function of the organism, experiments carried on over a period of some ten years by F.M. Pottenger, Jr. in U.S.A. become very relevant.[3] Working on experimental animals in connection with a Mental Hospital – following an accidental finding that cats kept on raw meat differed markedly in condition and were better subjects for operative procedures than those fed on cooked meat scraps from the Institution – he set up a series of feeding experiments to investigate the matter.

These were carried out in large cat pens (12 x 4 x 7ft.) kept out of doors each with a covered shelter at one end of the pen. The cats in four cages were fed separately. While on raw meat and raw milk both cats and their progeny were satisfactory in every way: they were in excellent condition. gentle in behaviour and free from disease. Those fed on cooked meat finished in poor condition, infested with intestinal parasites, had skin lesions and allergies, and were more difficult and often dangerous to handle. They reproduced poorly, were subject to abortion, inability to feed their offspring and produced malformed progeny. It took four generations of feeding on live food for them to recover from the defects and deficiencies once established in parent and progeny.

One significant comparison made by experiment was between cats fed on (i) raw milk; (ii) pasteurised milk; (iii) evaporated milk; (iv) sweetened condensed milk. Health was only sustained in the first of these cages. More was added to the above information. After the feeding experiments with the cats had come to an end, the pens were left fallow for some months. It was then noticed that weeds had grown in the pens but, though of the same kind, they were of very different growth and vigour. In the first pen (raw milk) they were flourishing. They diminished consecutively in (ii) and (iii), while in (iv) they were but poor and scanty in growth. Surprised by these findings, Pottenger sowed beans in all four cages. The result was that in (i) they grew flourishingly, climbing up the wire cage, while in other cages, like the weeds before them, they diminished in vigour consecutively, till in (iv) they made scarcely any growth at all.

These soils had been fertilised by the droppings and urine of the cats previously resident within each cage respectively. No other materials of any sort had been added to the soil in the cages.

This finding lends presumptive support to those who suspect that the nature of the farming procedures concerned with (1) the substances used in the fertilisation of the soil; (2) the feeding of beasts dunging the soil; (3) adjuvants administered to assist the breeding and rapid growth of young stock and the foreshortening of the reproductive cycle, can adversely affect the health of those fed on the produce of such husbandry. This question is applicable to the health and vitality of farm stock as well as to that of the human population. It is of maximum significance where the object of all farming is – or should be – the maintenance of human health.[4]

In view of the high incidence of degenerative diseases that now exists, attention to this subject would appear to be one of the first priorities in conservation of the physical and functional validity of the human in the process of ageing.

The nature of food is of critical importance for the elimination of disease, as was most dramatically demonstrated by the experiments of Major-General Sir Robert McCarrison while Director of the Nutritional Research Laboratory at Coonor in India.[5]

With long experience in the Indian Medical Service, McCarrison was struck by the very marked difference in stature, physical condition and vigour as well as in the incidence of disease in different races in India. He began to suspect that this was due to the difference in their traditional diets. In Coonor, he set up a series of experiments on rats to investigate this question.[6] The rats were housed in cages in the open air exposed to sunlight and fed on the full diets normally eaten by various races in India; e.g. Sikhs, Madrassis and Bengalis. The rats were kept under observation for 2½ years (i.e. the normal life span of the rat), after which time they were killed and a post-mortem examination made of all their organs.

The results were arresting. Those rats which had lived on the poorer diets, showed evidence of the diseases common to man; lung, intestinal, heart and kidney disorders being predominant among them. In the rats that had lived on the Sikh diet there was *no evidence of disease found*. Moreover, there had been deaths from disease in all other cages; but *no deaths* at all among those on the Sikh diet – except on the rare occasions in which an accident occurred to the offspring.

Astonishing as these findings were, they were even more significant when the circumstances in which the experiment had been conducted are closely examined. Coonor has what might be considered a perfect climate, temperate and equable, the temperature varying only a degree or two throughout the year. There was no shortage of labour for careful conduct of the experiments. One Sikh was employed for every eight cages for removal of the faeces, so that the possible contamination of the food should be reduced to a minimum; the food was all prepared and the green food grown on the site. The stock from which the rats were drawn consisted of some 1,000 rats or more consistently fed on Sikh diet. Among these also no deaths or disease occurred.

With masterly simplicity, though with scrupulous attention to experimental detail in conditions unparalleled perhaps in their suitability for experiment of this nature, McCarrison demonstrated experimentally, for the first time, the relation between diet and disease. More than this, he demonstrated that the organism can exist for its whole life span free from disease. Though the work of Weston Price, Wrench[7] and others have indicated that this can be true of man, it is not the common experience among civilised humans.

In looking at McCarrison's experiments from the viewpoint of their applicability to human beings, it is important to recognise the invariability of the conditions in which his rats existed. This was, indeed, one of the outstanding features of the work from the experimental point of view; one that makes it difficult to refute the evidence he produced. It has to be recognised that where human health is concerned we have to contend with the organism living *free* in its environment. Where the object is investigation into *health* rather than into the *absence of disease,* this introduces a further complication into all experimental procedures.

Adaptation

In all species living in freedom we are faced with what is termed 'adaptation of the organism to its environment'.

Where the one, viz. the environment, is fixed as in the case of the Coonor rats, there is little need for the exercise of 'adaptability' in the organism. While this is compatible with (physiological) 'existence', it is not compatible with the mutuality of synthesis between organism and environment in the actuality of *'living'*.[8]

Thirty years have passed since publication of the Cantor Lectures. Though McCarrison knew of the importance of adaptation as an aspect of nutrition, it necessarily remained a negative factor in experiments conducted in the conditions in which he was working.

Recently some interesting observations have been made by Dr. Crawford of the Nuffield Institute of Comparative Medicine, London Zoo[9], in comparing the nature of the tissue fatty acids of bovines in the wild with that of domestic cattle. Whereas the unsaturated or monosaturated fatty acids constituted some 30% in the wild animals, these are reduced to 2% of the total fatty acids in the domestic. As the unsaturated form is used in the structure of cell membranes – in particular in the endothelial cell membranes lining the arteries – this reduction may be of moment in human nutrition both in health, as well as in disease.

Additional evidence has been found by Dr. Sylvia Sikes[10] who, investigating the arterial system of elephants confined to the grasslands of a National Park, compared with elephants living free in woodlands on high ground, found that there is arterial disease in the former but none in the latter. While the latter live on oil-rich food, the former are confined to water-rich pastures. Here there would seem to be evidence of adaptation affecting the tissues of the body as well as the behaviour of the animals in domestication. It has been shown on the Haughley Research Farms that land fertilised with artificials yields products with a higher water content than the same products grown organically. In view of the fact that the populace in modern civilisation is living almost entirely on food grown with artificials, are humans being reduced to the same situation as elephants confined to the National Reserves and cattle fed on water-rich pastures?

That adaptive changes due to feeding affect the whole of the body tissues is no new finding. When considering utilisation in nutrition the work of Dr. Lionel Picton[11] is pertinent. He was one of the earliest and staunchest advocates of the importance of nutrition in the cultivation of health. His long experience in family practice, coupled with an exceptional power of observation, led him to realise the importance for good nutrition of the body of breast-feeding carried on till weaning was complete.

He shared this enthusiasm with the late Dr. Truby King who, after the first war, revived interest in breast-feeding among civilised peoples the world over. Dr. Picton relates[12] how the two friends were supping together at the same table as a Frenchman. Inevitably the two friends fell into a long discussion of the subject which interested them both so deeply. At last there came a pause. The Frenchman leaned forward. 'Messieurs, I am only a layman but I think I can corroborate all you say,' he said slightly to their surprise, 'I am a bootmaker in Paris. A gentleman comes into my shop wanting a pair of boots. I at once bring out for him the best I make. He is lost in admiration; such style, such cut; fine workmanship and fine leather. "How much?" Consternation! "Have you none less expensive?" "Mais oui, monsieur . . .", and I show him another pair. He looks enquiringly and then says ". . . but these look exactly the same, cut, style and finish and the price only one third that of the first pair. Why are the others so much more?"

'Then I tell him. "The first will grip your foot, keep their shape, the leather will not crack or lose its bloom and you will have them for years as good as new. Of the second pair I say, "you will be proud of them as you walk out of my shop; but in six months they will have lost their shape and a crackle will begin to appear all over the surface of the leather which will no longer take its original shine and soon you will have to discard them". Then I explain. "We

F

Parisiens, as you know, are very fond of our good veal. But to be good it must be veal of calves that have been fed naturally by their mothers. The first pair of boots I show you are made of the skin of those calves. The others, they are bucket-feds!".'

In this anecdote there is incontrovertible evidence that nutriment affects the texture of the whole body. Dr. Picton reinforces this by reference to the rashers of bacon which used to be open to the housewife's inspection on the grocer's counter. One lot will be of consistently firm texture, the fat lying close up against the lean without interruption. Another batch will show moist fat of differing texture beneath the rind, than a line of fascia, loose and separated from both fat and lean. The first will be from young pigs that have been running with the sow for 10 or even 12 weeks; the second from piglets removed from the mother at 6-8 weeks; both pigs finally, of course, having reached the approved *weight* for slaughter. He goes on to say that even if the piglets in the last few weeks are only allowed to suckle once a day, this will prevent the change in appearance of the flesh on slaughter.

But there are many factors which, at present, we do not understand. *How* food is utilised appears, then, to be of some consequence.

Cleave and Campbell[13] in their book on the saccharine diseases demonstrate that the saccharine substances are not partially distributed in the body destroying only the teeth – which we can see and feel, or raising the blood-sugar content – which we can measure. *All* the *tissues* are affected by the relatively unaccustomed intake; though some organs are slower to show signs of the strain and injury imposed upon them.

These workers, moreover, show that the way in which such substances are ingested and digested is of·critical importance; rapid influx into the body of 'pure', refined carbohydrates does great harm, while the same quantity, unrefined and combined with cruder matter and therefore ingested at a slower rate, can even be beneficial. Quantity multiplied by time is a factor in utilisation.

Moreover, not all persons respond to the insult (damage) of inappropriate food such as refined carbohydrates in the same way, as Cleave and Campbell point out; some show relatively early, others much later (20 years), others not at all. The vagary of symptomatology is attributed to 'personal build'[14] which renders some more open to the manifestation of symptoms than others. While recognising this factor as 'hereditary', they insist that it is not one due to a genetic hereditary defect.

That there are factors of 'hereditary' origin which are not genetic agrees with my own experience while working with families under continuous observation in Peckham. So impressed were we with the evidence, that we have come to speak of, and work on, the basis of a dual inheritance of the child; (i) a *genetic inheritance;* (ii) a *nurtural inheritance*[15].

The genetic inheritance we see as the inherent *specific content* of the new individual with its chromosome endowment – a mutualised contribution from male and female parents. Whereas the nurtural inheritance is the *specific context* of the new individual conceived within the body of the mother whose specific constitution has already been tinctured with the specificity of her male. This context extends after birth to cover the parental 'home'. This is the position of organism when seen as an ecological entity defined in terms of functional action.

Recognition of these two 'inheritable' factors, both acquired from the parents, serve to emphasise the uniqueness of the individual dependant not only upon his specific genetic endowment, but also subject to the inescapable influence of the ecological locus he acquires at conception and occupies at least up till birth.

No doubt some 'advanced' thinkers hurrying to get rid of this nurtural inheritance – 'accident of birth' and stigma of circumstance – would hail the possibility of test-tube births for this reason. But the practical necessity, as Cleave and Campbell say, of emphasising the distinction between the two factors and of recognising them as given bionomic features in the make-up of each personality, is great. In humans relatively little can be done about genetic inheritance, (except in disease) but much can be done about the circumstances that determine the nurtural inheritance where there is knowledge; and, I would add, the will to effect change. This is clear from what we have seen above of the 'adaptability' of the organism to its environment.

Some Conditions Associated with Nutrition in the Embryo[16]

There is a question that never ceases to baffle us: if nutrition can alter the very tissues of the body, how is the uniqueness of the individuality sustained? On this matter I propose to offer some observations arising out of certain anatomical dispositions in the development of the embryo.

Fortunately natural circumstances have provided a perfect demonstration-preparation of some features of the nutritional process in the early stages of development of the individual. Something as commonplace as the hen's egg will serve as an example for our purpose.

Within the shell of a fertilised egg – perhaps nowadays not so commonplace an object – lies the ovum provided with the total nutrient material required for its growth into a live chick. Let us then take a look at what is inside this egg: and also examine what goes on as the chick is growing the structure and organs of its body.

Inside the germ-cell is the chick's genetic inheritance – its complement of chromosomes which is a dual contribution from its parents. This genetic endowment ensures to it, before development gets under way, a bi-polar basis of male and female bias for each step in its coming growth programme. The factor of bi-polarity, apart from that of sex bias, is one common to all functional action in health[17] although it is not one to which any importance has so far been attributed.

Before fertilisation occurs the germ-cell has already collected from the tissue fluids of the maternal ovary of its origin a relatively huge supply of provender – the yellow of the egg – a contribution to the chick's development before it is hatched. This yolk material is enclosed in a membrane, the yolk-sac lodged within the germ-cell. This membrane expands like a balloon on the surface of which the small ovum lies.

Wrapped around the germ-cell – but entirely *outside it* – is the 'white' of the egg. This is a secretion poured out from the lining cells of the maternal oviduct while the egg is on the way to the nest. The germ-cell equipped with all its nutrient supplies for the growth of the chick, is now sealed up in the shell. Nothing more will be added till hatching has occurred.

The 'white' included within the shell by the hen is a *parental* contribution to the ovum. It is a complicated albuminous substance of highly specific pattern – that of the specificity of the parents. It is not, however, of a pattern wholly 'foreign' to the ovum, for it is of the same pattern of specificity as the tissue fluids of the maternal ovary in which the germ-cell was immersed while collecting its yolk substance before fertilisation. These tissue fluids of the hen had already been attuned to the specificity of the cock by the absorption of the testicular products at the time of conjugation. The 'white' therefore is a substance bearing a *group-specific* pattern common to both parent and offspring. Nonetheless it is still outside the body of the ovum; it has not yet been 'accepted' by it and become of the 'self' stamped with the new entity's own personal pattern of specificity.

Attention must now be given to what happens as the ovum grows within the shell up to the time of hatching. Gradually both sources of nutrient material are used up; that which was outside the ovum and that which was inside disappear. In due time from within an empty shell there steps out a live chick. A marvel of bionomic synthesis has occurred; nothing has been added; and nothing rejected and there has been no waste!

The progressive stages of development within the shell as the two nutrients have mingled and become converted into the chick, merit close study and cannot be dealt with here. But the significant feature in the process is the very early formation of blood channels in association with the yolk-sac membrane. These develop into the vitelline vessels of the developing chick, so linking the material in the yolk-sac with the systematic vessels soon to develop in the body of the growing embryo and through which the substance of the 'white' is transported for utilisation within. This makes possible from the beginning of development a continuous intermingling of the contents of the yolk-sac with the incoming material of the 'white' from outside the ovum.

Within the yolk-sac membrane inside the ovum the 'yellow' of the egg, already of the 'self' with its unique constitution, is thus in a position to act as template, or guide, to the pattern of specificity to which the newly entering material from the outside must conform in participating in the synthesis which is to produce the body of the unique chick.

Mammalian Development

In the development of the mammal a great step forward has been taken in the early process of nutrition. The developing chick in the avian egg has to rely till hatching on food laid down before its growth begins; and so is reared on preserved food. But in the mammal provision is made for the young embryo to carry on its earliest exercise in synthesis on fresh, up-to-date material. This been achieved by the ovum being implanted in the maternal womb before any development begins, the nutrient supplies from the beginning being drawn from the mother's blood. They are adjusted to the minute to minute changes in the ecological locus of the growing individual.

In mammalian development, where no time is lost in the

76

fertilised ovum becoming implanted in the womb, there is no need for the accumulation of any large store of personal supplies to last till hatching occurs, so no yolk-sac forms before implantation. Nevertheless the yolk-sac principle is by no means discarded; for no sooner is the ovum implanted in the womb than a relatively small and flaccid sac (the secondary yolk-sac) appears within it. Up till now the embryologist, believing this structure serves no functional purpose, has disregarded its significance.

The transient appearance of this structure within the mammalian ovum might indeed easily cause it to be so disregarded were it not that soon some remarkable happenings can be observed. In the mesenthelial tissue intervening between the yolk-sac membrane and the slender body of the developing ovum, blood-lakes begin to appear. These go on to form, as in the chick embryo, the *first* communicating blood channels within the developing embryo. As in the avian egg, again these turn into the vitelline vessels of the embryo. In the mammalian embryo they link up with the systematic vessels forming later to convey nutrients from the placenta to the body of the embryo. As in the chick embryo there is this early blending of what has been secreted by the ovum and is already of the 'self' and that not yet of the 'self' which is brought in from the outside.

Nowadays we are familiar with synthesis of proteins according to specific patterns induced through nuclear and cytoplasmic elements in the cells. Circumstances which would make such a process possible are here seen as already present for the earliest steps in synthesis in the embryo.

But this is not all. By the time only a few of the body cells stretching from head to tail of the embryo have been laid down, the membrane of the yolk-sac proceeds to throw out membranous prolongations along the ventral surface of this embryonic body throughout its length, finally coming to line the cavity of the archenteron, or what was formerly called the fore, mid and hind gut.

We must accept this membrane of the yolk-sac as the structure that carries the *function* of the sac, for it was this layer of cells that was initially responsible for secretion of the yolk-substance into the sac. As embryonic growth proceeds the archenteron, the embryonic structure that this membrane comes to line, becomes the alimentary canal with its associated organs such as thyroid, thymus, liver, pancreas, etc., that develop from the gut wall providing later *internal* secretions into the adult body.

No sooner has the yolk-sac membrane been securely incorporated into the body structure, than the embryo in its growth encircles and constricts the neck of the sac which consequently shrivels and disappears.

So though the yolk-sac has vanished before birth, by that time its secreting membrane is firmly lodged within the adult body. Here then the membrane and the structures that have developed from it are in a position to continue to produce secretions capable of acting as templates of the specific pattern of the 'self' in all syntheses which nutrition in the individual demands. By this means the progressive individualisation of the entity can be sustained within the dictates of its genetic inheritance.

Should the function of a personal yolk-sac prove to be part of the essential equipment for the nutritional process in health, where we are to look for it in the adult body of the organism into which the yolk-sac derivates have been incorporated? Furthermore, how are we to recognise its special contribution from the 'self' (i.e. from *within* the body), to full functional action in the nutritional field? These are questions which arose out of the Peckham Experiment; they await future experimental confirmation. But we suspect they are deeply involved in the process of utilisation.

Some indications as to where it might be useful to pursue the search for an answer to the first question will be found in the chapter on Aesthesia in *Science, Synthesis and Sanity* where the proposition of an *aesthetico-directive system* within the adult body is put forward.[18] In health we see this system as operating from *within* in unity of functional action with the well recognised and deeply explored sensory-motor system that responds to environmental impacts deriving from *without*.

This would mean that the organism functioning in health proceeds on a bi-polar basis – from *within – out* and from *without – in*. Such a provision would allow the organism to sustain its ecological poise in mutuality – in the process of its growth, and maintain its unique individuality in face of the unceasing shifts in its ecological locus.

But leaving aside a subject perhaps too abstruse for our purpose at this moment, we can nonetheless recognise from the earliest stages in the nutritional process the provision existing in the organism for a function that relates heterologous patterns of specificity from the outside to the 'self'. Recent attempts at surgical introduction of foreign tissues and organs into the body have emphasised the importance of the existence of such a function.

The New Born

It is not surprising to find that at birth provision for the next stage in development of the individual has followed the same principle. In the course of advance in evolutionary development, the free moving young of the mammal released from the womb have been provided with breast-milk for their first nutritional excursion after birth.

To understand the full significance of this, we must go back once more to foetal life and ask what the foetus is doing while in the womb? It is busy elaborating the structures of its body – the *organic mechanism,* or tools, with which it will have to live. By the time of birth these anatomical features are complete; head, eyes, ears, limbs, internal organs, brain, communicating vessels . . . all are there. But few, other than the heart, have been put to any use; the legs cannot walk, the eyes cannot see, nor the lungs breath. The *capacity* for action is there; but the *capability* to do has yet to be learned.

The ability to use any one of the capacities for which the young are structurally endowed at birth follows a very definite pattern – sudden desire to do the thing; the almost instant ability to do it on broad lines of achievement; the persistent eager repetition of action once acquired over a period usually covering some weeks; followed by the sudden cessation of interest in the action in favour of the next achievement. This process in relation to the finer co-ordinations in the development of the young child was first described by Maria Montessori. Later it was studied by us in the Pioneer Health Centre for the grosser co-ordinated actions of children up to puberty and after the war in the infant from birth onwards.[19]

The outstanding feature of the process is the child's sudden spontaneous eagerness to do and to pursue a particular action, its unmistakeable pleasure in doing it, and subsequent satisfaction in the achievement. For these reasons we have called such incidents in behaviour *appetitive phases;* these phases cover a spontaneous primary facultisation of capacities hitherto unused.

There seems to be as definite a succession in functional development, i.e. in the spontaneous use of the capacities latent in the anatomical structures and organs of the body between birth and puberty as there is known to be a consistent sequence in the development of the organs and structures in embryonic life. There is a rich field for future experiment in this subject.[20]

In the new born child the all important development of the capacity for primary use of the alimentary canal is well exemplified. In this process the appetitive phase for learning is readily recognisable – sudden desire to find the breast, insistent attempts to suck, eager repetition of these actions with increasing proficiency in doing so effectively; complete concentration on the process and the obvious satisfaction in achievement.

The above sequence of events we found in the breast-fed babies of which we had an unusually high proportion in Peckham. In these babies, who with their mothers were in very full health, establishment on the breast took an average of not less than 6-8 weeks. That is to say it takes not less than six weeks for the baby to become adept in the use of its alimentary apparatus with its first food after birth. The outstanding aspect of these babies was one of serenity; their gain was steady and not too great, their digestion smooth and untroubled, sleep regular and almost continuous till establishment and the bowel action regular and inoffensive. Abdominal upsets, allergies, rashes and other disturbances were rarely if ever met with and there was seldom any prolonged crying.[21]

In health, the foetus grows spontaneously and in ease in the womb, so it should not surprise us that the infant at birth should continue to do likewise when taking advantage of the provision nature has made for it. But this of course will only be the case where the mother functioning in health is, so to speak, biologically valid and free from major defects and deficiencies.

We are usually told the only unreproducible advantage of breast milk is the protective substances it provides in the colostrum not easily reproduced in processed or manufactured forms of infant food. The baby at first is, however, not merely 'feeding', i.e. supplying itself with the substance for growth and arming itself with temporary protection from certain infections. It has to learn *how* to metabolise the nutrients to fit its own unique pattern of action. Instead of a substance totally unknown the newborn is offered for its first exercise in the functional action of its gut, something of a group-specific pattern that it already knows; something in quality like that which it has been accustomed to. Breast-milk is a parental contribution to its nutrition in a sense parallel to the 'white' of the egg contributed to the growing chick within the egg shell. It is a substance tempered to its capacity for learning the 'how' of metabolising the food intake from outside to fit the needs of the unique constitution of the learner.

Deprived of their mother's milk the bucket-feds' build bodies of but poor quality. Could it be that the structure of the organic mechanism is degraded as a result of by-passing the patterns of specificity in the materials used in first steps in synthesis? Is it a matter of how the immature learn to build their bodies? Have we hit on *how* the difference arose in the Frenchman's two pairs of boots?

There is a question of great significance here. Does *how* the infant learns the first steps in the process of metabolism influence the way it will tend to carry on its metabolic processes throughout life? Does the initial mode of learning influence how it will be enabled to meet the challenge of insults – nutritional and infective – as and when they come upon it throughout life? *Is this learning essential to the laying down of the mode of action that underlies health?*

When the adult is faced with increasing age and loses some of the powers of compensation so abundant in youth, there is a tendency to revert to habits, metabolic and others – acquired in childhood. When disease intervenes, do we see here in retrospect an inadequate method of metabolism learnt in infancy? Or again, where inadequate provision of food has led to defective offspring born of deficient parents, does the inability of the next generation to learn efficient means of metabolism in infancy explain the three generations or more of adequate feeding it takes to regain full health in the offspring?

In brief, is the use of a 'blue print' for instruction as to *how* to build in the specific pattern of its own unique personality as necessary for the new-born as it is for the foetus in the womb? Is this where the foundations of health lie?

So in full swing we come round to social implications of deep moment. If the early developing embryo learns *how* to utilise the food available to it – through the medium of a group-specific substance deriving from its parents – then it would appear that evolution maintains the distinction of the species by sustaining what we have called the *nurtural inheritance* of the individual.

In that case the notion of 'family' exerting its inherent capacity for parenthood no longer appears as a mere 'cultural' institution to be accepted, or rejected according to political persuasion, or fashion. It rises into prominence as a biological necessity in the full functional development of all the more highly differentiated species in the scale of evolution.

References

1. This book has been out of print since Weston Price's death. It is now in the course of republication and to be had from Price-Pottenger Foundation Inc., 137, No. Canyon Blvd., Monrovia, California, 91016.
2. Schneider, Howard A. Institute for Biomedical Research, Education and Research Foundation, American Medical Association, Chicago, Illinois. 182nd Scientific Meeting Lecture, Royal Veterinary College, London, 22nd July, 1966.
3. Pottenger, Francis, K. Jr. The effect of Heat Processed foods and metabolized Vitamin D Milk on the Dentofacial structures of experimental animals. *American Journal of Orthodontics and Oral Surgery,* Vol. 32, No. 8. *Oral Surgery,* pages 467-485. August, 1946. Obtainable from Price-Pottenger Foundation Inc., 137, No. Canyon Blvd., Monrovia, California, 91016.
4. Robb, Lindsay. Agriculture and Medicine. *Guy's Hospital Gazette,* 20th July, 1968.
5. Sinclair, H.M. (Editor). *The Work of Sir Robert McCarrison,* Faber and Faber, 1953.
6. McCarrison, Maj.-Gen. Sir Robert. *Nutrition and National Health* (Cantor Lectures), Faber and Faber, 1945.
7. Wrench, G.T. *The Wheel of Health.* The C.W. Daniel Company Ltd., London, 1938.
8. Williamson, G.S. & Pearse, I.H. *Science, Synthesis and Sanity* (Chap. I). Collins, London, 1965.
9. Crawford, M.A., Gale, M.M., Woodford, M.H. & Casper, N.M. *Int, Jour. Biochem.,* Vol. 1, No. 3. June, 1970.

10. Sikes, Sylvia K. Observations on the Ecology of Arterial Disease in the African Elephant (Loxodonta Africana) in Kenya and Uganda. *Symp. zool. Soc. Lond.* (1968) No. 21, 251-273.
11. Picton, Lionel James. *Thoughts on Feeding,* Faber and Faber, 1946.
12. *ibid.,* p. 102.
13. Cleave, T.L. & Campbell, G.D. *Diabetes, Coronary Thrombosis and the Saccharine Disease.* John Wright & Sons, Bristol, 1966.
14. *ibid.,* p. 3.
15. *Science, Synthesis and Sanity,* pp. 137-138, 249.
16. *ibid.* See Chap. VIII, 'Internal Faculties'.
17. *ibid.* See Chap. IX, 'Bipolarity in Facultisation'.
18. *ibid.,* pp. 208-213.
19. In preparation by I.H. Pearse.
20. Pearse, I.H., & Crocker, Lucy H., *The Peckham Experiment,* George Allen & Unwin, London, 1943, pp. 182-183.
21. *ibid.,* p. 171.

5. Modern diet and degenerative diseases

Professor Hugh Sinclair

Dr. Sinclair is Fellow of Magdalen College, University of Oxford, and Visiting Professor of Food Science in the University of Reading. He believes that an excess of saturated fatty acids and a deficiency of essential ones in our diet as a result of changes in animal feeds and food processing is leading to a fault in our cell structure which predisposes us to many diseases.

The following is taken from a tape-recording of an unscripted talk.

WHEN I was a medical student just before the war, I noticed what lots of other people have noticed, but no-one seems to have thought very much about, namely that the expectation of life of a middle-aged man has hardly changed over the last hundred years. Now this, I think, is the most interesting single fact in medicine today, that a little over a hundred years ago a middle-aged man could expect to live almost as long in this country as a middle-aged man can expect to live today. The precise figures are 20 years in 1841 and 23.2 years in 1963. We have very good mortality figures for middle-aged men and others from the 1840s. There was a careful statistician – William Farr – who collected, for the first time, accurate statistics and published them, and, if we look at his tables with reference to what middle-aged men or others were dying of a hundred years ago, we find it was largely due to infections. By far the most important causes of death were pneumonia and tuberculosis – and there were many other infections, including typhoid and typhus. In Oxford there was a cholera epidemic in 1854, but at that time the chronic degenerative diseases such as heart disease and forms of cancer were rarely recorded. I do not want to dwell on the one or two possible minor fallacies in these statistics. Of course, many cases of heart disease must have been missed and put down to other causes; for instance there was a cause of death 'ague' that occurred in the tables which does not occur today. And certainly there were mis-diagnoses, but, in general, the statistics relating to cancer could be generally regarded as a correct indication.

Indeed, there is a variety of evidence to show that the chronic degenerative diseases have, in countries such as the U.K., been rising very rapidly since those days and it so happens that as such diseases – say coronary heart disease – have been rising, the infections have been falling. The infections, of course, have been falling because of the widespread use in the last few decades of antibiotics. In the U.K. during the last two decades, pneumonia has become quite unimportant and so has tuberculosis. However, it is now predicted by the statisticians that the expectation of life of middle-aged men will actually now fall in this country, because the incidence of chronic degenerative diseases is increasing very rapdily, and at the same time it appears that the base line in the infections has been reached.

Almost every major advance in medicine has occurred over the last few decades – a hundred and thirty years ago there were virtually none of the drugs we use today, only opium and its derivatives, and, of course, no endocrine preparations, no insulin, no liver therapy, no vitamins, none of the great advances, and, of course, no antiseptic surgery and no anaesthetics – they came in about a century ago. So despite all the great advances, it would appear that we can do little about the chronic degenerative diseases which are going on increasing very rapidly. And if this is so, there must be a reason, there must be something changing in our environment which is having this dramatic effect upon our health. I thought as a student this was the most interesting thing in medicine to study. I came to the conclusion that this change in disease pattern must be linked to a change in nutrition. Of course, various things like diesel fumes and stress have been incriminated, that I am perfectly prepared to discuss, but I think they are secondary or unimportant.

If, over the last 100 years, there has been a change in our food going on, then what type of change could it be? Even as a medical student I thought the two things that were most likely to be changing were the fats in our diet and the trace elements. That is to say, these are the two changes most likely to produce this tremendous rise in chronic degenerative diseases. In 1937, just after I had qualified in medicine, I went to the United States to see the work then being done on what are called the essential fatty acids, the fats we must have in our diet in order to keep healthy. It was obvious to me that there were several ways of looking at this general nutritional problem. One is the longitudinal approach over the years, and there is also the entirely different cross-sectional approach – that is to say, what is happening at a given time: say, at the present time, in different countries or in different people in one country who eat differently. Thirdly, there is another approach, nothing like so important, but relevant: namely, what happens in lower animals under domestication rather than in their natural habitat. A fourth approach is purely experimental in which one observes the effects of different diets deliberately fed to animals and/or man.

Taking the longitudinal approach, we find that there are a number of different chronic degenerative diseases that are increasing at roughly the same rate in countries such as this, but which are rare in underprivileged countries. Until 1926, coronary heart disease was rarely recorded. Sir John McNee, a distinguished doctor living in Hampshire in 1925 published, in a British medical journal, two cases of coronary heart disease which he happened to have seen in the United States. This was obviously considered a rare condition. Today, we may have two cases coming into hospital daily. So this cannot be due only to electrocardiographs helping

G

with more fashionable diagnosis. There is a great deal of statistical evidence that the incidence of the condition must have been rising. A very interesting point is that when the second world war started this rise stopped and there was even perhaps a slight fall. This pattern occurred in all age groups. Then, in 1943, the rise was resumed – although the war continued for two more years. It also appears that there was a little drop in '48 and another in '53, since when the rise has continued. Let us take an entirely different disease in which the diagnosis is unmistakeable, perforated duodenal ulcers. Professor Illingworth's figures show that the pattern of incidence is very roughly the same, except that a sudden peak in duodenal ulcers appeared in 1940 and 1941 at the start of the war and then duodenal ulcers went up at a similar rate to coronaries. Another disease that has been rapidly increasing is slipped intervertebral discs. Mr. Laurence Knights mentions appendicitis and gall-stones. I would like to mention another entirely different disease, called senile osteoporosis, i.e. fractures of the neck of the femur; again, an unmistakeable diagnosis. These fractures of the neck of the femur are increasing very rapidly. Mr. Knights will bear me out in saying that, in general, these fractures are not primarily due to people slipping on icy streets, or some other kind of accident trauma. There is something fundamentally wrong with the connective tissues of the bone – it's not demineralisation, it's not calcium lack, it's the protein matrix of the bone, that is the connective tissue which is disordered. So here we have very different diseases, all linked together on a degenerative basis.

Can we in any way relate these very different diseases, together with a number of others, all of which are increasing at a similar rate in the U.K. (and which are rare in underprivileged countries)? Can we relate them to diet?

Here I must say just a little about fats, because I think these are one of the main things we have to consider. In general we can divide fats into two different types which in very loose terms we can call 'useful' and 'harmful'.

'Useful' because there are certain fats which we must have in the diet as the body needs them for particular purposes and cannot make them. If the body is to get them, they have to come from the diet. Opposing these are the fatty acids which the body can make, for instance from carbohydrate. We believe, or most of us believe, the main reason why we need the essential fats is that they are essential constituents of the cell membranes and intracellular structures. These essential fatty acids have a peculiar structure, curved round, and in membranes they form 'bricks' of a very particular shape. If there is an excess of the wrong type of fat, it will become incorporated into the cell membrane and make it unstable – this can be shown very easily by experimental work on animals. The animal looks quite normal but is very susceptible to a whole variety of insults, whereas animals fed with other essential fatty acids will withstand such insults. This is really what one would expect. If one thought of building cell membranes like building a house, the bricklayer would want bricks of various particular sizes and shapes to put into his wall to make them fit together. If he were provided with an excessive quantity of bricks of the wrong shape he might use them, but the wall he would then build would have neither the required symmetry nor shape, nor strength. Turning this analogy to the build-up of cell membranes, if they are faultily built they can be very easily disrupted. It is for this reason, in my view, that a very different pattern of diseases can be produced by the same basic fault. Take, for instance, one that I have not mentioned, poliomyelitis, a disease of the nervous system. It is well known that poliomyelitis is very much commoner in privileged countries than in under-privileged countries. The orthodox explanation of this is that in under-privileged countries hygiene is bad, so the children get small doses of the polio virus when they are young and so they become immune. In lower animals it can be shown that if the cell membrane is faulty in structure there is vastly increased permeability which means that viruses, bacteria and toxic substances might get in more easily. For this reason we find that infants or lower animals that are deficient in essential fatty acids are much more susceptible to infections. This fault, and its relations to the mitochrondia (a sort of energy storehouse of the cell) could be extremely relevant to cancer. Many years ago when I was working with an Indian professor, we showed that animals deficient in essential fatty acids were much more susceptible to a substance that produces cancer. This could be relevant to lung cancer. But what is absolutely certain is that this is not the whole explanation. I've been in Japan, where statistics for this disease are published, and I've also collected figures from Spain, where there are no published figures, and these show, in both countries, that lung cancer is a comparatively rare disease. But smoking is extremely prevalent. In Japan they even smoke the last bits of cigarettes off a pin to get the entire satisfaction. In the U.K. the incidence of lung cancer is going up much more quickly than is smoking. It is much too much a male disease here. Women, 20 years ago, were smoking a lot of cigarettes and yet still lung cancer in this country is a rare disease in women as compared with men.

This difference between men and women is an important one. You may have wondered why I emphasised the level of expectation of life of middle-aged men. Many of the degenerative diseases are some ten times commoner in middle-aged men than women. Take coronary thrombosis, for instance, which in middle-age is ten times commoner in men; for lung cancer the ratio is very much greater than that. We can show in lower animals that their requirement of essential fatty acids is ten times greater in male animals than in females during the period of reproductive life. You may wonder about the differences noted at the beginning of World War II, when perforated duodenal ulcers shot up in men and then resumed the ordinary curve, while coronaries stopped rising. It is possible that duodenal ulcers are caused by a faulty membranous lining to the duodenum and that this fault is made evident when hydrochloric acid from the stomach is poured onto it. That is to say, a healthy duodemun would withstand much hydrochloric acid from the stomach, but if this structural defect is present then ulceration results. It is a well-known fact that more hydrochloric acid is put out under conditions of stress such as during war, so that this increase highlights faults in the duodenal mucosa caused by faulty diet.

What about coronaries? Perhaps this is the most interesting disease of all. Its incidence in Scandinavian countries is similar to that seen in this country, so it is clearly not an artefact of diagnosis and it is clearly not due to fewer doctors being about during the war. Various people have said that with the onset of war when we had petrol rationing people took more exercise, so there were then fewer coronaries. Various people have said that stress causes coronaries – less stress, less coronaries! Although I believe stress is a factor in this, I think the most important factor is a dietary change. In 1943, when the war continued and petrol rationing continued, coronaries suddenly started to go up when we had a dramatic change in our diet. The changes centred largely on three foodstuffs from America, hydrogenated margarine, very fat bacon which is saturated fat and a tinned meat that is rich in saturated fat. These suddenly came into our diet.

I have collected the figures from chronic schizophrenics in mental hospitals in Britain before, during and after the second world war, because these chronic schizophrenics in mental hospitals did not know there was a war on. They were not affected by petrol rationing or by extra stress – but with them, so far as I can see, their pattern of degenerative diseases followed roughly the pattern already described. The one thing that affected the chronic schizophrenic that affected us in the same way was the change in their food.

And, finally, these findings have been subsequently confirmed in lower animals, under different circumstances and experimentally produced alterations. Some very interesting work has been done recently in the Nuffield Department of Comparative Medicine at the Zoo in London. We had a symposium there about a year ago on coronary thrombosis and athero-sclerosis (1968, *Symp. Zool. Soc. Lond. 21*), in animals of all different sorts. For instance, it was shown that elephants in Africa don't have much of the type of fats which cause athero-sclerosis in the blood vessels, but elephants in the zoo had; and this is, in general, true in most animals. Thus, if they have to eat our diet, these animals get our diseases. And we can, of course, produce these diseases in lower animals by putting them on the wrong type of fats. Three very important experiments have been done, two of exceptional importance, of taking middle-aged men and, with their consent, altering their diet. Dr. Leren in Norway and Dr. Turpeinen in Finland have done this in rather different ways and run their experiments for 10 years. What Dr. Leren did was to take middle-aged men who had had a coronary, wait one year and then divide them at random with their full consent, into two groups, altering the fats in the diet of one of them and not in the other. Then, following them for five years, he found that by this alteration in fat, that is, by replacing harmful fats (normally predominating in Western diets) by useful fats he significantly reduced deaths from second coronaries. Dr. Turpeinen followed a different path; he took chronic schizophrenics in two mental hospitals in Finland and divided them into two groups. They were absolutely healthy except for their schizophrenia – no high blood pressure, none of them had any heart trouble, and so forth. And he altered the fats in one group and not in the other. Let me say at once that this is an absolutely ethical, experiment; the consent of the mental patients means absolutely nothing, but here he was *improving* the diet of one group and keeping the other on their normal diet, an absolutely ethical thing to do. In the group in which he improved the fats by increasing the essential fatty acids, keeping the carbohydrates the same, keeping the sugar the same, keeping the calories the same, the proteins the same, everything except the quality of the fat, he also got a significant reduction in deaths from the first coronary.

How have we been changing our diets so that the essential fatty acids have fallen and the saturated fatty acids have risen? In fatty acids there are carbon atoms which can be either joined by a single link, with carbon having four bonds on it, or they can be joined by two links – two bonds joining the carbon atoms together – and this is called un-saturated; it's called unsaturated because other atoms can be added. Suffice to say that the unsaturated ones are unstable, because if they take up oxygen they become rancid and toxic. So the food manufacturer very properly wants to get rid of them, because he does not want rancid fats about, he wants the stable ones. It is these essential fatty acids which are the basis of the drying oils in paints. You all know that if you open a tin of paint, which has linseed oil in it, one of the unstable fats, a skin forms on the top of the paint where the air is in contact which means that oxygen is taken up, converting these highly unstable liquid fats into solid saturated fats; that is what the skin is on top of paint, and that is what drying oils are. The margarine manufacturer has to make oils more solid which he does by hydrogenating – putting hydrogen onto the double bonds I described. A leading firm has introduced a margarine called 'Flora' which has 50% of this type of fat in it, which is an excellent amount – this will be a very important change for the good in our diet. So the food manufacturer can, and will, do quite a lot.

I can give an example of a fat with which we are all familiar, namely lard, pork fat. Until about 1939, pigs used to be free ranging and producing soft fat on them. Then it appears that policy decreed that the public wanted hard fat on bacon. So now all pigs are produced to have hard fat by feeding them on carbohydrates, and, further, there has been another complete change in lard. Housewives will remember that before the war lard used to be bought from a butcher who rendered it down each day, and if it went rancid in a couple of days, he threw it away. It was rich in the most useful type of fat and if it went rancid it lost them. Now, of course, you can't buy lard from a butcher, you buy it from a grocer or a supermarket. It's in a package. You can't put something in a packet which is going to go rancid in a couple of days. It's got to have a shelf life of months. Therefore, it is hydrogenated. So here is a complete difference. And of course chicken's eggs are going the same way as is most of our food – hens fed on stable foods – and stable, containing saturated fat, means that the animal has the wrong type of fat; therefore when we eat the animal it has this wrong type of fat rather than the fat we really want. Thus, there has been a very undesirable change going on in our fats in recent years.

The main difficulty in improving diet is the amazing lack of research in human nutrition. The first thing we need is the facts – and facts can only be got by research, whether it is epidemiological research, which includes following patterns of disease in different countries, or in one country over years, or whether it is experimental research, doing experiments on man or on lower animals. Just to give you one example, in 1946 my university was offered a large sum of money for founding an Institute of Human Nutrition. But the university turned it down, since it was believed that after ten years had passed from the cessation of World War II, there would be no human nutritional problems to study! After having worked under primitive conditions for ten years, I thought of going to the States; then Lord Woolton lent his support to the establishment of a National Institute of Human Nutrition.

Plans are now being made to set this up as an International Institute of Human Nutrition, with similar Institutes in other countries since the problems of human nutrition are world-wide. Such an Institute should have a first class library and should do broadly based experimental work as well as gathering facts from different countries together. The late Sir Robert McCarrison gave me his personal library because he was very interested in setting up this type of Institute. At the moment this is in store waiting for a building to put it all in, and, in addition, I have a fine collection of nutritional books and journals as well as

70,000 reprints. If funds were available such an Institute could start in the immediate future near Oxford.

6. White bread and brown in relation to nutritional deficiencies

S.J.L. Mount, B.A., M.B., M.R.C.P., D.C.H.

Dr. Mount adds further evidence of the effects of refined carbo-hydrates on health. Formerly Secretary of the McCarrison Society, he has made a special study of this subject.

> There was a jolly miller once
> Lived by the river Dee,
> He worked and sang from morn till night
> No lark more blithe than he.
> And this the burden of his song
> Forever used to be,
> I care for nobody no not I,
> And nobody cares for me.

WHAT was true two hundred years ago is true today. The miller is concerned to sell his wares. If it is easier to mill white flour, bake white flour and sell white flour, then white flour will be sold. 'The consumer is king' is the cry. 'Let the consumer choose. Let others concern themselves with health and leave the miller alone! If the public want white bread, they shall have white bread'; and so the story goes on.

Unfortunately (for the nutritionist) it appears that the public do prefer white bread, *if not educated otherwise.* During the last war, for political and economic reasons, flour of coarser extraction was enforced. Many found that the bread made from this flour was tastier and more whole-some than the finer white product. However, in many of us, there linger subtle desires that are not easily assuaged. White denotes purity. Smoothness of texture is pleasant to the tongue. Smooth white bread tastes 'nice'; it is a 'delicate' food. Smooth fine light white bread soon appears superior to her coarser and darker cousin. Modern television advertisements associate white bread with feather-light young girls that float up in the air in balloons!

History shows that these tendencies have been with us for many years. In Leviticus there is the reference 'He shall bring for his offering the tenth part of an ephah of fine flour' (Leviticus 5:11). The Greeks regarded black bread as the food of common use. The Egyptians also prized white flour. It is well to remember however that fine flour in ancient times was stone ground and more cream in colour than white. Wheat germ gave white flour its creamy colour and in the mid-nineteenth century mills (steel mills) were invented that could extract wheat germ from the white starchy endosperm. Herein lies the problem, for in aiming for a whiter flour the miller had to exclude the richest nutritional part of the grain – the germ – from the final product.

The germ of wheat is that part of the seed that surrounds the plumule and radicle. It will feed the new shoots when the seed germinates in the ground. It is therefore rich in vitamins, protein, and fat. The minerals reside for the most part in the aleurone, one of the outer layers of the wheat grain which are lost in milling. The germ however contains most of the B vitamins, most of the essential fats of the grain and carries a better quality of protein into the bargain. Dismiss the germ and you exclude the heart of the grain. Unfortunately, however, germ-rich flour is oily, stores badly and can go rancid. Hence another advantage to the miller. If the germ was excluded from the flour, the flour then kept better! Economic forces are stronger than altruistic health considerations, and by the end of the nineteenth century refined wheat flour was in common use throughout the country. The position is unchanged today.

What however is changed today is our overall nutritional

intake. Technology has altered our environment. Food is processed in new ways: the consumption of bread and the nutritional importance of bread has to be viewed against this changed setting. So much of our food is subject to softening, refining, processing and remixing that a protest movement against such measures is growing. A section of the population is beginning to complain about its bread. The fine white flour of Leviticus has now been baked into a limp and tasteless offering, which surely any high priest would reject! A century ago bread was the staple food of the lower classes. It is unlikely that any class could now sustain its strength and health on our contemporary product.

Bread consumption is falling and has been falling for forty years. Bread now contributes only 15% of our calories and 13% of our calcium. Not long ago it contributed 30% to our national calorie intake and a good quantity of our vitamins. Meat, milk and flour are our three nutritional mainstays today and flour (bread, pastry, cake and biscuit) contributes 27% of our calories, 26% of our protein, 28% of our thiamine, supposedly 27% of our iron, 23% of our nicotinic acid, 20% of our calcium and 5% of our riboflavin. We should look therefore at our nutritional intake of such vitamins, minerals, protein and fibre as are contained in flour: then we should look to see if deficiencies occurring in the population can be correlated with nutrient abstractions from flour.

Protein

Milk and eggs have a higher quality protein than wheat flour. Wheat flour protein is low in essential amino acids, lysine and tryptophane. Wholemeal bread however contains more lysine than refined white bread as the germ in wholemeal bread is richer in lysine. Our protein intake in western countries is large enough and varied enough to exclude this as an advantage. McCance and Widdowson and also McCarrison have shown that refined flour is less effective in promoting growth of weanling rats than wholemeal flour where the diet contains flour as the main source of protein.

Vitamins

Wholemeal bread of 90% – 100% extraction contains a vastly greater concentration of B vitamins than refined white bread. Table 1 shows the drastic drop that occurs in flour on refining. Table 2 shows the amount of vitamins by percentage that are lost by this technological process. Cereals are an important source of all B vitamins, including the lesser known ones such as inositol, para amino benzoic acid, biotin and pyridoxin. If these are whittled away out of our diet by refining, there is a possibility that nutritional deficiencies will arise.

As regards the four lesser known B vitamins, mentioned above, very little is known as regards man's exact requirements. Little is known either concerning his intake. H.M. Sinclair has argued that pyridoxin deficiency is probable as a consequence of refining processes and this may contribute to the presence of arteriosclerosis in man. But these are little explored areas of nutritional health and one has to pass over them in search of more definite data. Suffice it to say that ignorance is no justification for confidence.

Folic acid, a B vitamin depleted considerably in the milling process of flour, is now recognised as deficient in the blood stream of 25% of women in pregnancy in this country. Folic acid is found in green vegetables and cereals and cereals are an important source of the vitamin as the cooking of vegetables destroys folic acid. Deficiency of this vitamin has been shown to occur in a multitude of experiments concerning pregnant women and it has also been shown to be deficient in old people, especially those who live alone. In old people it merely leads to anaemia: in pregnancy its reactions are more sinister as it produces abortions and congenital malformations. Wholemeal flour contains far more folic acid than refined flour, and is vital in this respect to the maintenance of full health.

There is no concrete evidence, at the present time, of clinical thiamine, riboflavin or nicotinic acid deficiency amongst the general population. Marginal and submarginal vitamin states are hard to assess and define and this aspect of vitamin nutrition has yet to be researched. It would seem possible from food intake studies, however, that a certain segment of the population is sailing close to the wind. The three groups particularly at risk, who have been shown to take an inadequate diet under certain circumstances, are the elderly, the young and teenagers. Children nowadays are brought up in an environment permeated with destructive enticements. Lollipops, ice cream, sweets and crisps can all contribute to lowering a child's nutritional status. Dr. G. Lynch and Dr. Sylvia de la Paz of the Social Nutrition Research Unit of Queen Elizabeth College, London, have recently reported that two thirds of the country's school children in England and Wales eat unsatisfactorily. Emphasis is laid by these research workers on the detrimental role played by the school tuck shops in this respect which can so easily entice children away from sound food and school meals. Dr. G. Taylor has outlined in his turn the clinical evidence for vitamin deficiency in the elderly. The evidence suggests that vitamin intakes are suffering in these groups. It remains to follow up the survey work with biochemical assessments.

The refining of flour, by depleting bread and flour products of B vitamins, could contribute to national nutritional deficiency. Of the vitamins removed but two are synthetically replaced – thiamine and nicotinic acid – and this only in half measure and only in bread.

Vitamin E

Vitamin E is destroyed in refined white flour. Chlorine dioxide, the bleacher commonly used in milling, destroys the vitamin E content of flour, which is reduced anyway by the milling process. Accurate vitamin E needs have not been assessed for man, but wholemeal flour represents one of the richest sources of this vitamin. Vitamin E is a mysterious factor, which has yet really to prove itself in the service of man. Rats need it and chicks need it, but man is an elusive animal to pin down in the laboratory and scientists are undecided yet as to how necessary it is for humans. Vitamin deficiency states can arise in man as anaemia following certain diseases of the intestine such as steattorrhoea.

Essential Fats

Certain oils are essential to man. These are unsaturated in their hydrogen content and number amongst them such fatty acids as linoleic, linolenic and arachadonic acids. They are found in higher concentration in wholemeal bread than refined white bread, in fact their concentration in the latter foodstuff is very low as chlorine dioxide, again acting detrimentally, tends to cause saturation of the double bond. This changes the nature of the fat from soft to hard. However, flour is not an important source of essential fatty acids (providing some 2g daily out of a possible 14g intake) and the nutritional damage following consumption of white flour in this respect is probably small.

Minerals

Wholemeal bread is richer in calcium, sodium, potassium, magnesium, manganese, iron, copper, phosphorus and sulphur than refined white bread. It is also richer in trace elements arsenic, iodine, bromine, cobalt, lithium, titanium, nickel, aluminium, tin and silver. Very little is known concerning trace element nutrition in man and this area must remain a silent area for the time being. Certain evidence brought together by Schroeder in America confirms that wholemeal cereals are important as a rich source of trace minerals in the diet, as are fresh vegetables, fruit and pulses: but how these factors affect man's health must remain pure speculation at the present time. It would seem that trace element nutrition will become more important as the years go by. Schroeder makes the point that as food is processed and refined, trace element loss is increased. Fresh fruit and vegetables, wholegrain cereals and sea food are the richest sources of trace elements in our diet. Less and less of these foods are being eaten at the present time. We are living in times of great change. These changes are bound to affect our health in many and various ways.

For many years it has been the custom of orthodox nutritionists to pooh-pooh wholemeal bread. In support of this they argue that the phytate content of wholemeal bread is a disadvantage to the human body as this compound forms an insoluble complex with calcium in the gut (and with iron too) and so depletes the body of this mineral rather than building up its absorbtion. Scientific research is equivocal on this issue. Walker has shown that the body, given time enough (up to six months), adapts to high phytate intake and achieves calcium balance on varied diets. McCance in early studies, but taken over a short term, showed calcium depletion following phytate ingestion. Widdowson in certain experiments carried out in Germany in 1951 showed later that humans react in a diverse and varied manner to phytate ingestion, so no firm rules could be laid down as to how much phytate should or should not be consumed. Many other factors affect calcium absorbtion besides phytic acid and these include vitamin D content of the diet, total amount of calcium consumed, season of the year, period of time over which the diet is consumed and degree of malnutrition and health in the subject. It is highly unlikely that in a healthy western diet any subject would deplete his body of calcium by eating wholemeal bread. The argument becomes even less convincing when it is realised that bread constitutes on the average but 15% of our national calorie intake, and wholemeal bread is a certain source of many minerals of value to the human body, not least magnesium. Other minerals of obvious value have been mentioned above and include phosphorus, sulphur, copper and iron.

Fibre

One of the greatest advantages held by wholemeal bread is its content of fibre. One hundred per cent wholemeal bread is rich in this factor. More and more food is consumed nowadays after refining and diets generally are soft, pappy and fibreless. Complications are inevitable at a certain stage. The peristalsis of the intestine is dependent upon the bulk of food and the nature of the bulk. If fibre is lacking from food the mass of intestinal contents is prone to form a dense bolus of putty like nature. This cannot be propelled along the intestinal tract with the same ease as a fibre-rich bolus. Constipation is but one of the hazards that follows. Haemorrhoids, diverticulitis and appendicitis are other diseases associated with chronic constipation. Chronic constipation itself cannot be recommended, though many of us suffer a mild degree of this! Bowel evacuations take place twice a day on a fibre-rich diet and the time food takes to pass through the intestine is halved. A soft diet may take 34 hours in passage, a fibre-rich diet 15 hours. Bowel evacuation is also more complete on the latter diet.

Cleave in his contribution to this book brings forward convincing evidence for the association of diverticulitis, appendicitis, haemorrhoids, varicose veins, cholecystitis, urinary infections, renal stones, diabetes, heart disease and obesity with the consumption of white refined flour and sugar in a modern diet. Dental caries is a more obvious example still where sticky carbohydrate foods such as biscuits predispose to the development of tooth decay. Experiments show that a refined soft diet in which white flour replaces wholemeal flour predisposes to dental caries. Sugar is of course also a primary factor in the aetiology of this disease.

Apart from these important considerations of the part played by fibre, research has also indicated that particular factors reside in wholemeal bread that have a special and directed effect in preventing dental caries. The factors appear to be linked with the phosphate and with the

H

phytate in wholemeal. It is quite possible that other factors which have specific nutritional advantages reside in natural foodstuffs and are undiscovered as yet. Schneider has shown by careful and painstaking work that whole wheat carries certain factors which he terms pacifarms. These give mice the ability to resist salmonella infection. They are destroyed by milling. Nutrition is a relatively undeveloped science and much remains to be discovered. It would be shortsighted to deny this and claim that the laboratory bench had at this stage revealed all that is contained within our food.

Additives and Chemicals in Bread

The following additives are associated with bread making:

Bleaching and Improving Agents
chlorine dioxide
potassium bromate
ammonium or potassium persulphate
benzoyl peroxide
chlorine (cake flours)
sulphur dioxide (biscuits)

Emulsifying Agents
super glycerinated fats
stearyl tartrate
lecithin

Preservatives
propionic acid
calcium or sodium propionate
acetic acid
mono calcium phosphate

Most of these chemicals have been officially cleared as safe in breadmaking processes by such national bodies as the Food Standards Committee. Most of the compounds have been toxicologically tested in the laboratory. But as scientists now admit this type of testing is not a complete safeguard to health. No food additive is ever absolutely safe. We are besieged by such a multitude of additives and food chemicals in our diet that it is impossible for any scientists, or any scientific body for that matter, to clear all as safe, for the interactions and possible combinations between chemicals are so many in number. Any one of these interactions could theoretically be toxic. We are in the 'hands of the gods', and there seems little we can do about it except eat raw food, natural foodstuffs and wholefood! This would appear reasonable in the circumstances, in view of the traps and pitfalls laid by modern technological processes.

Experiments in a German orphanage

In the final analysis it is not what food contains but how it affects our total health that matters. Professor McCance and co-workers after the last war carried out researches on children in German orphanages that had far-reaching effects; for they showed that over the eighteen months of the experiment, no definite health advantage seemed to follow from the consumption of wholemeal bread as compared to 70% extraction rate refined white bread. It is worthwhile to examine this experiment in detail as it holds such an important place in nutritional research concerning bread.

Three hundred and ten boys and girls from two orphanages took part. They were split into five sections according to the type of bread eaten:

1. Those eating 100% wholemeal bread
2.   ,,   ,,   85% refined flour bread
3.   ,,   ,,   70%   ,,   ,,   ,,   unenriched
4.   ,,   ,,   70%   ,,   ,,   ,,   enriched to the
                    100% level
5.   ,,   ,,   refined flour bread enriched to the
                    85% level

Enrichment involved the addition of thiamine, nicotinic acid, riboflavin, iron and calcium.

The diet was 70% of bread, 21% of vegetable and

4% of milk. Supplements of vitamins A, D and C were given all children. The experiment was therefore to test the sufficiency of the supply of B vitamins, minerals and protein from different breads. Biochemical estimations were made of vitamin concentrations in the blood and excretion from the body.

All children were found to improve in health. As war orphanage children, they had been subsisting on a very poor quality diet and were found to be suffering from a variety of skin conditions together with poor stature. The conditions of the experiment provided them with good vitamin supplements of vitamins A, D and C, a lot of protein, as they could eat unlimited bread, and more calories than they had ever consumed before. It would have been remarkable if their general nutrition had not improved!

What is important for our purposes, however, is to compare the total nutrition of these children with that often found amongst contemporary British children. The orphanage diet was plain and simple and calorie intake at one orphanage, as has been quoted, was derived 70% from bread, 21% from vegetables and 4% from milk. The orphanage children were therefore vegetarian and consumed a fair quantity of vegetables both root and leaf. The vegetable water was always conserved for making soup, and must have supplied a fair amount of minerals and trace elements. Children nowadays often consume little in the way of fresh vegetable or fresh vegetable soup, and tend to fill up on snacks, lollipops, ice cream, sweets and crisps!

The German experiment is not relevant to children with a belly full of snacks, crisps and sweet consumption, who cannot afford to lower general vitamin and mineral intake beyond a certain point. This point has been reached. Many children in the contemporary situation are taking in submarginal amounts of vitamins and general nutrients, and so exist below this cut-off level. They are existing therefore on a poorer diet than the orphanage children in the experiment, a diet far higher in its content of sugar and refined foods.

Dr. Lynch and Dr. de la Paz in their examination of the diets of 4,000 children in England and Wales found that 33% of children were eating an insufficient and poorly nourishing diet. This was due to a number of factors which included breakfasts that were skimped, school tuck shops that prevented children from taking school lunches and poor value evening meals when parents were away from home. Lower standards were found in the south-east of England where only 28% of children were taking a satisfactory diet. In the north of England the figure rose to 46%. If this is a true situation it is a drastic one.

On this evidence it is deplorable that bread is eaten in the refined white state. We should be especially concerned over the long term effects of this subnutrition. More and more food nowadays is processed and the lack of fibre can cause serious intestinal diseases later in life. This has already been discussed. We seem therefore to have moved in the past 100 years from an undersupply of the right foods to an overabundance of the wrong ones and it is our children that will suffer for this. Now is the time to put this situation right.

The nutritional arguments that support the production of true 97% – 100% wholemeal bread within the context of modern living and sophisticated food consumption are overwhelming. It would be folly to ignore them. The human body is not infinitely adaptable, and it is unwise to think it is.

TABLE 1. *Nutritional composition of wholemeal and 70% enriched white bread*

Nutrient	mg per 100 g	
	Wholemeal Bread	White Bread
Vitamins		
Thiamine	0.2	0.18
Riboflavin	0.1	—
Nicotinic acid	3.5	1.7
Pyridoxine	0.5	0.15
Pantothenic acid*	0.8	0.34
Biotin*	0.007	0.0008
Folic acid*	0.026	0.014
Linoleic	800	530
Tocopherol	2.2	0.85
Minerals		
Sodium	466	515
Potassium	261	106
Calcium	26	92
Magnesium	89	22.6
Manganese	2.4	0.3
Iron	2.8	.1.8
Copper	0.46	0.13
Phosphorus	240	81
Sulphur	81	77

Other minerals contained in whole wheat flour:
Arsenic, Iodine, Bromine, Cobalt, Lithium, Titanium, Nickel, Aluminium, Tin, Silver.

*Figures taken from Kent-Jones D.W. and Sinclair H.M. All other figures taken from McCance R.A. and Widdowson B.M.: The Composition of Foods, H.M.S.O. 1960.

TABLE 2. Proportion of certain vitamins lost in the milling of 70% extraction flour

Vitamins	Percent loss
Pyridoxine	84
Biotin	77
Folic acid	68
Riboflavin	67
Pantothenic acid	50
Thiamine	80 (40% after replacement)
Nicotinic	77 (40% after replacement)
Vitamin E	100*

*Vitamin E is lost through milling and destroyed by chlorine dioxide.

Source: Moran T. (1959) *Nutr. Abst. and Reviews 29, 1.*

7. Nutritional deficiencies in elderly people in western countries

Geoffrey Taylor, M.A., M.B., (Camb.), M.R.C.P. (Lond.)

Returning from many years work in eastern countries, Dr. Taylor was surprised to find signs of classical nutritional deficiencies in people of all ages in this country. He explains why he thinks this is happening.

THE study of nutritional deficiencies in elderly people is important for several reasons. The health of the elderly may be improved, and the study may throw light on possible nutritional defects, which have begun earlier in life. Possible nutritional factors may be found, causing such common diseases as gastric ulcer, diverticulitis, varicose veins, diabetes and even coronary thrombosis and strokes. Elderly people in hospital can be studied for long periods on a known hospital diet.

I am neither a trained nutritionalist nor a geriatric physician. I have worked for over 20 years in India and Pakistan in the Indian Medical Service, where as Professor of Medicine at Lahore, and Consultant Physician to the 14th Army, the study of nutrition was obviously a most important part of the teaching and practice of medicine.

Sir Robert McCarrison by his work relating different physiques and diseases of Indian peoples to varying diets[1], had a great influence on medicine in India, as elsewhere. In the Punjab, for example, medical students were taught that the so-called diseases of civilisation, gastro-intestinal diseases, such as gastric ulcer, appendicitis, diverticulitis, dental caries, coronary thrombosis and diabetes, were rare or even non-existent in village Punjabis, while they lived in their own villages, eating their traditional diet of chappati (whole wheat flour), dhall (peas and lentils), lhasi and dhai (milk curds), some vegetables, and occasionally meat. When Punjabis migrated to Indian cities and changed their diet to a Westernised one, they tended to have a similar incidence of these diseases as we do in western countries. Perhaps the most striking example was with dental caries. The teeth of the village Punjabis were excellent, with an exceptionally low caries rate, but in the children of middle class Punjabis in Lahore, who tended to eat sugar and sweets and the refined carbohydrates of western countries, caries was often as common as in Britain.

I also had the opportunity of studying conditions in severe famines, in the South Russian Famine in the early '30s, in the Punjab Hissar Famine in the late '30s, and finally in the Bengal Famine in 1943, where I had direct responsibility for starving and grossly malnourished patients.

Returning to Britain, I was surprised to find signs of classical nutritional deficiencies in many people of all ages, especially in the elderly. I have been fortunate in being able to study these in over 50 hospitals and in six nutritional surveys during the last five years. I was obviously influenced by work in India, again especially by Sir Robert McCarrison. Recently in Britain, Surgeon-Captain Cleave, and his colleagues in their book on saccharine disease[2] have given further evidence supporting that of Sir Robert McCarrison.

After the Second World War, for the last 20 years, there have been repeated yearly reassurances by Ministers of Health that apart from exceptional cases, there were no appreciable nutritional deficiencies in Britain. These reassurances were based on the Annual Report of the National Food Survey Committee and reports of general and geriatric physicians, that they were finding few or no signs of nutritional defects.

There was therefore considerable surprise in the mid '60s when four surveys[3,4,5,6], of vitamin C levels in elderly people showed a majority of elderly people in hospitals to have very low levels of vitamin C in the blood, that they were below the levels of elderly people living at home, and that these levels fell the longer they were in hospital.

These findings should not have been surprising because Professor Platt in 1963[7] had shown that most of the vitamin C in hospital and institutional diets is destroyed in all but small hospitals. His report showed that mass cooking for over 50 people in hospitals, canteens, schools and other institutions, including meals on wheels, often destroys up to 90% of the vitamin C in the food.

Working as a locum consultant physician I was able to begin nutritional trials in hospitals at Cheltenham and Yeovil, giving supplements of the B group of vitamins and vitamin C to elderly patients for periods up to a year. These patients had classical signs of malnutrition in their lips, tongue and skin. I found, as I had previously found in India and Pakistan, that these signs tended to disappear with nutritional supplements. I concluded therefore that elderly people in Britain are often suffering from nutritional deficiencies both in and out of hospital.

The World Health Organisation[8] summarises the present knowledge of these conditions. In recent work I have been doing, I have paid special attention to the following conditions:–

Angular-stomatitis, a condition with cracks or fissures at the angles of the mouth, with sodden, pale epithelium-cheilosis, fissuring or cracking of the lips, with redness, swelling or ulceration, with pale, sodden epithelium-glossitis, a term used for lesions on the upper surface of the tongue, which may be a brighter red than normal, with white swollen filiform papillae (these cover the upper surface of the tongue and are normally pink) which may be partly or completely shed, leaving a bare tongue. Other papillae, the fungiform papillae, may be enlarged and red: cracks or fissures may appear – nasio-labial dyssebacea, a condition of the nasio-labial fold, in which the glands enlarge and become red with scaliness of the skin. These conditions may be present in varying degrees and stages, involving only the tip or margin of the tongue. The United States Nutritional Survey in 1963 states that 'the presence of moderate degrees of atrophy of the filiform papillae, fissures, redness or magenta coloured tongue, *even in a small percentage* of a population is highly suggestive of a deficiency of some members of the B complex (B12, Folacin, Niacin, B6 or of iron)'.

Five years ago, while working in a hospital at Kettering. I observed in the tongue of an old man the onset of acute sub-lingual haemorrhages, and was able to photograph them. Petechial (sub-lingual) haemorrhages were followed a week later by generalised haemorrhages on his lips and mouth. on the skin and into his joints. The saturated vitamin C test in the urine was very prolonged and he had a history of non-existent vitamin C in his diet. There were no other positive findings. A diagnosis of acute scurvy was made. These acute petechial haemorrhages on the under surface of the tongue, were related to a general red increase and dilatation of small blood vessels (vascularisation), with blurred edges and apparently red varices, and older blue varices. Some of these dilatations appeared to be small micro-aneurysms. Photographs of the under surface of the tongue made possible a careful study and record of these changes. These conditions were described in acute scurvy 400 years ago, and by Lind over 200 years ago[9]. I was thus led to examine many thousands of mainly old people during the last five years. I have concluded that in Britain 90% of patients in most hospitals show these changes and that 80% of elderly people outside hospital also have them. They appear in some young people in the early '20s whose diet is low in vitamin C.

Recently in acute scurvy developing experimentally in American prisoners in civilian jails[10], similar dilatation of vessels and micro-aneurysms have been observed and photographed in the eye. Similar eye changes occur in elderly people in Britain.

Experimental work in guinea pigs with acute scurvy show slowing of the circulation, dilatation of small blood vessels and haemorrhages caused by slight trauma. Sections of these conditions show dilatation of small vessels with red blood cells outside the vessel wall, confirming what is seen in the photographs.

A recent paper by Windsor and Williams[11] suggests that collagen metabolism is impaired in patients with levels of vitamin C four or five times the level at which acute scurvy is developed. An earlier paper[12] on experimental scurvy in guinea pigs shows that if guinea pigs recover from one attack of acute scurvy, they develop a second attack after four or five days of a scorbutic diet, instead of 24 or 25 days needed for the first attack. If these two observations are related, they may explain why up to 90% of elderly people in British hospitals have these sub-lingual conditions. In the Farnborough Survey described in more detail later, over 60% of patients had vitamin C levels below that suggested by Windsor and Williams to cause damage to collagen and fibrous tissue formation.

These sub-lingual changes possibly related to low vitamin C levels are almost certainly world-wide in both developed and under-developed countries. I have seen sub-lingual haemorrhages and varices commonly in elderly people in one Austrian hospital, and in young and middle-aged German workers in a Dusseldorf steel factory. A paper from the Indian Nutrition Research Laboratories[13] shows that the levels of ascorbic acid in leucocytes in well-to-do and poorer Indian peoples, and in Indian pregnant women and children in South India, are much below the level which Windsor and Williams consider necessary to prevent disordered collagen metabolism and defective fibrous tissue formation.

At the end of 1965 a 'double blind' therapeutic trial[14] was organised in four South London hospitals on 80 elderly patients, to attempt to assess the effects of vitamin supplements (B group vitamins and vitamin C). Forty patients were given large doses of the B group of vitamins and vitamin C (Thiamine 15 mg, Riboflavin 15 mg, Nicotinamide 50 mg, Pyrodoxine 10 mg, and Ascorbic Acid 200 mg.), the other 40 being given placebo tablets with no vitamin content. The untreated group showed clinical evidence of deterioration, especially during illnesses, when they were treated with anti-biotics. The treated group showed clinical and biochemical evidence of marked improvement. I was responsible for the clinical examinations which I did every three months. I also photographed the lips, the upper and lower surface of the tongue and the skin. At the end of a year I was able to decide which cases had had active tablets and which had had dummy ones, with only one mistake, by observing the improvement or deterioration in the lips, tongue, skin, eyes and the general mental and physical conditions, including the number of skin haemorrhages ('senile purpura'), the Hess test, and myoedema (myotatic irritability). Looking back with hindsight, it was possible to show that these changes could have been seen at three months. I was especially impressed by the general improvement in mental and physical conditions, as well as the improvement in the physical signs. One important finding was that bedsores in the treated group tended to recover, in the untreated group they became worse.

When the year's trial was finished the vitamin supplements were stopped. Within six months, on a hospital diet without supplements, the original classical signs of malnutrition returned. In some cases these signs were more marked than at the beginning of the trial.

This Farnborough trial is important because it establishes that the so-called classical signs of malnutrition are present very commonly in elderly patients in British hospitals; in fact only four out of the 80 patients were graded as normal at the beginning of the trial. It is perhaps significant that the hospital food in these four hospitals was thought to be some of the best in British hospitals.

The mucous membrane of the mouth and tongue, which can so easily be observed and photographed, has for many years been regarded as indicating the state of the gastro-intestinal tract, a 'raw red tongue indicates a raw red gut' is an old medical aphorism. Recent biochemistry suggests that the state of the cells of the mucous membrane of the tongue and mouth is similar to all other cells in the body. They show visually, without recourse to endoscopy or surgery, the first clinical signs of nutritional or metabolic disorders. Photographs give a permanent record.

These signs in the mouth and tongue may be related to other diseases as McCarrison taught many years ago. Recently work in Glasgow[15] has shown that symptoms and bleeding from gastro-intestinal lesions are related to low vitamin C levels. Surgeon-Captain Cleave and his colleagues are suggesting that the changes in diet of the last 100 years may be also related to many of the common diseases in Britain. Perhaps the most striking aspect of the Farnborough trial was the great improvement in the mental as well as the general physical conditions of patients getting vitamin supplements. There is some evidence[16] which suggests that atheroma (thickening of the arteries) begins with tiny haemorrhages related to low vitamin C levels in the wall of blood vessels, similar to those which are observed on the under surface of the tongue.

The Farnborough trial has been followed by several others. It was necessary to find whether the signs observed in hospital patients occurred in elderly people, living at home, who were not sick. Under the auspices of the Royal College of General Practitioners, a survey of 217 elderly patients on doctors' lists were surveyed. A high incidence of epithelial and vascular lesions of the tongue and skin, which had been shown in the Farnborough trial to respond to treatment with the B group of vitamins and vitamin C, were observed. Only 20% were graded as normal. The paper on this is due for publication shortly[17]. These signs were advanced in most cases and indicate that they had been present for many years, beginning in middle life, or earlier. The signs were more common in men than in women, they were related to social class, smoking, peptic ulcer, and frequency of consumption of vegetables and fruit. They were not related to age, or living alone. The signs were more common in social classes 4 and 5, unskilled or semi-skilled workers and their wives.

During the survey, it was found that many housewives often over-cook green vegetables or add soda to them during cooking, destroying the vitamin C content. For example, in Swansea in 18 out of the 20 households visited, soda was added to cabbage or brussels sprouts. The Opinion Research Centre hearing of these findings, recently (1970) did a nation-wide survey[18] and found that 27% of British housewives still add soda to green vegetables. This percentage varies with social class, and in different parts of the country. For example, this addition of soda is much more prevalent in households of unskilled or semi-skilled workers and in large industrial towns. In the Midlands, for example, 45% of housewives add soda to their green vegetables. These rather surprising findings, together with the work of Windsor and Williams, show that the estimate of the vitamin C content of British diets made by the National Food Survey Committee needs re-consideration as no account of this destruction by soda of vitamin C is taken in these official estimates.

Three other surveys are due to be finished in 1970 or early 1971. The Department of Health and Social Security asked me to take part in a trial in five London hospitals using vitamin supplements. Another trial with individual vitamins is being completed in South London, and a third trial in Edinburgh is endeavouring to assess mental and physical improvement or deterioration with or without vitamin supplements.

Whatever the result of these trials, at least it is now clear that the so-called classical signs of malnutrition are very common in elderly people in Britain and that they begin often at quite an early age.

As the result of more detailed large photographs of the tongue, and with the assistance of Dr. Murray, Director of the Mycology Department of London School of Hygiene and Tropical Medicine, the Department of Health trial has established that fungus infections (candida) of the elderly are very common both in hospital patients, and in elderly people outside hospital, that these candida infections may be related to malnutrition, infection and anti-biotic treatment, especially tetracycline. Further work is needed to determine the significance of this finding.

Many questions arise from this evidence. At what age do these defects begin? What effect have they on the health and efficiency of people in Britain, in the developed countries with similar diets and with similar signs in underdeveloped countries? What relation have they to such diseases as gastric ulcer, gastro-intestinal haemorrhage, diverticulitis, strokes, heart failures, coronary disease, hypothermia, arthritis, bedsores, and to the ageing process itself, and how can they be prevented?

There is now enough evidence to warrant the immediate setting up of a new clinical research unit, preferably in a teaching hospital, to investigate these nutritional problems, using new biochemical and other new techniques. For example, there has not been until recently a reliable biochemical technique to estimate riboflavin, and the methods of estimating vitamin C and vitamin B1 are difficult and often not standardised, the results from one laboratory not being related to those of another.

The changes in British diet during the last 100 years are described elsewhere in this symposium. It is important, however, to recall that in 1956 the war-time flour was changed to a whiter flour, 30% being removed and used for animal feeding. This 30% contained most of the roughage and iron, the B group of vitamins and calcium of the wheat grain. Because of this it was decided in 1956, to reinforce white flour with iron, calcium, vitamin B1 and nicotinic acid. Work mainly by Elwood summarised in *Iron in Flour*[19] shows that the iron added to white flour is poorly absorbed and has little effect on haemoglobin levels. More recent work shows that iron is more readily absorbed from whole wheat flour than from the present 70% extraction white flour. Iron must still be added by law to white flour in Britain, although Elwood's work has shown it is of little use. His work is an interesting example of the complexity of modern nutritional problems and the need for more exact research.

The study of vitamin deficiencies is obviously only a small part of the nutritional work needed. Obesity for example is obvious to anyone who uses his or her eyes. Probably 50% of adult British people are overweight and at least 20% of children. Children's teeth are increasingly carious, mainly because of excessive sugar, sweets and refined carbohydrates. Osteo-porosis is very common in all elderly people. There is evidence to suggest that part of the cause may be low calcium intake in our diet and low vitamin D levels. The need for urgent research is obvious.

There are powerful vested interests to preserve present conditions and resist, perhaps unconsciously, change or recognition of nutritional defects. The vast interests concerned with sugar, white flour, fat, meat and butter are some of the most powerful. For example, if excessive saturated fat in our diets is found to be one of the factors causing thickened arteries, leading to heart attacks and strokes, the consumption of saturated fats should surely decrease in the near future. Butter, olive oil and ground-nut oil are mainly saturated fats. We are told there are 'mountains' of butter unsold in Europe, olive oil is a major product in Southern Europe, and ground-nuts a main crop in Africa. To change from mainly saturated to unsaturated fats in our diet, which may be necessary, will therefore involve vast changes in agriculture, as well as in the food industry generally.

Associated therefore with a new clinical research unit, a publicity organisation is needed to inform the public of new findings, and suggest how changes in diet can most easily be made. The experience of the failure of the anti-smoking campaign during the last 15 years illustrates the power of vested interests coupled with public apathy and conservatism.

119

Until more knowledge is available, it is possible to make definite suggestions to improve nutrition. Until hospital diets can be improved there is a need for vitamin supplements of the B group of vitamins, vitamin C and vitamins A and D, particularly for elderly people in long stay hospitals. Obviously we need publicity to stop the addition of soda to green vegetables when they are cooked. We need publicity to suggest that green vegetables should be cooked for not more than five minutes or so, that they should be served immediately after cooking. We need propaganda to increase the regular eating of more fruit and green vegetables and the cutting out of eating sweets and excessive quantities of sugar. We need to know the present evidence of the relationship between saturated fats and thickening of the arteries and whether to eat the present amounts of butter, cream and animal fats.

The immediate problem is to get something done on a national scale in the next year or two. I suggest therefore that the British Nutrition Foundation brings together representatives from the Royal College of Physicians, the Royal College of General Practitioners, the British Medical Association and the Medical Research Council to sift the present evidence of malnutrition in Britain and to set up a new Clinical Nutrition Research Unit. I suggest that it is now urgent to reconsider whether the British recommended levels of vitamins and other nutrients in food need revision, and whether a change in the Government policy on the present '30% extraction' white flour is needed.

References

1. McCarrison R. and Sinclair H.M. (1953) *Nutrition and Health*, Faber & Faber.
2. Cleave T.L., Campbell G.D., and Painter N.S. *Diabetes, Coronary Thrombosis and the Saccharine Disease*, 2nd Edition, 1969, J. Wright & Son, Bristol.
3. Bowers E.F. and Kubik M.M. (1965) *Brit. J. Clin. Pract.* 19, 141.

4. Kataria M.S. *et al.* (1965) *Geront-Clin.* (Basle), 7, 189.

5. Griffiths L.L. *et al.* (1967) *Geront-Clin.* (Basle), 9, 1.

6. Griffiths L.L. *et al.* (1968) *Geront-Clin.* (Basle), 10, 309.

7. Platt B.S., Eddy T.P. and Pellett P.L. *Food in hospitals,* Oxford Univ. Press, Oxford 1963.

8. World Health Organisation. Expert Committee on Medical Assessment of Nutritional Status 1963, W.H.O. Technical Report Series No. 258.

9. Lind J. (1753) *A treatise of the scurvy,* 1st Edition. Reprinted in 1953 – edited by Stewart G.P. and Guthrie D. Edinburgh Univ. Press.

10. Hood J., Hodges R.E. (1969) *Am. J. Clin. Nut.,* 22, 5, 559.

11. Windsor A.C.M. and Williams C.B. (1970) *Brit. Med. J. I.,* 732.

12. Mounquand G., Michel P. and Bernhein (1924). *Acad. de Sci.* Vol. 176, p. 1655 and in Monograph of the Pickett Thomson Research Lab. Vol I. Sept. 1931 *The Vitamins.* E. Brownings, published by Brailliere Tindall & Cox.

13. Mohanram M. (1965) *Ind. Jour. Med. Res.,* 53, 9.

14. Exton-Smith A.N., and Scott D.L. *Vitamins in the Elderly,* 1968. J. Wright & Son, Bristol.

15. Dymock I.W. *et al.* (1967) *Brit. Med. J.,* May 6, 375.

16. Sokoloff B. *et al.* (1966) *Jour. Am. Geriatric Soc.,* 14, No. 12, 123 q.

17. *Journal of the Royal College of General Practitioners,* May, 1971.

18. Opinion Research Centre, 47 Victoria Street, London S.W.1. (1970) *The use of Bicarbonate in Cooking.*

19. *Iron in Flour* (1968) H.M.S.O.

8. Some hazards of present day diet

Laurence E.D. Knights, F.R.C.S.

Working as a surgeon in Sierra Leone, Mr. Knights realised that he seldom or never operated on patients who were suffering from the diseases that occupied most of his working time in England. On returning home he set out to discover why this was the case.

I AM A general surgeon, interested in making people well. Sometimes, as for example in the case of injury, this wish is realised and patients restored to anatomical and functional normality. Two-thirds of my work is not of this nature. It consists of extirpation of tissues so damaged that they are a threat to well-being or to life itself. This damage is, I believe, for the most part, due to the food we eat, or the air we breathe, or to toxic substances we introduce into our bodies with the blessing of the Ministry concerned or, on occasion, of that of the medical profession.

Nutrition I would like to define, not in medical dictionary terms, namely the process of assimilating food because that process seems to me to be covered by digestion and metabolism. When we say food is nutritious, we mean that it is good for you, so human nutrition is concerned with the factors making for perfect functioning of tissues and bodily systems, with resultant health of mind and body. Impairment of nutrition results in an unnatural awareness of our body functions, a vague unease which may eventually culminate in a clinically definable disease process.

The *Medical News* recently carried an intriguing article

on the Tarahumara Indians who live 'in the rugged, forbidding mountains of northern Mexico, at an altitude of 8,000 ft. and are generally as unhealthy as any uncivilised people but who can run like hell'. Dr. Dale Groom, a cardiologist, states that their physical endurance and cardiovascular response are truly amazing. Almost from birth, the Tarahumaras, both male and female, engage in long-distance 'kickball' running. They kick a ball carved from a tree, the size of a tennis ball, tremendous distances, sometimes more than 100 miles. These long-distance races were a national sport. There are about 50,000 Tarahumaras and the various tribes compete periodically and bet on the outcome. Dr. Groom examined them before and after they had run a race of nearly 29 miles for his benefit. Electrocardiograms were completely normal, he said, and chest x-rays showed normal heart sizes, even in Indians who had been running long distances for many years. He notes that this is contrary to the oft-cited enlargement of the athlete's heart. At the end of a race, they showed very little rise of pulse rate and were not even winded, though they had each lost about 5 lb. in weight. These Indians, he said, often hunted for meat by literally running a deer to death. Ranch owners in areas abutting the mountainous region occasionally hired Tarahumaras to chase and catch wild horses.

A further note of the Tarahumaras, kindly supplied by Mr. Leonard S. Zahn, states:

'The Tarahumaras would be considered malnourished by most criteria. Infant mortality is very high – only the fittest survive. Their teeth appear good. They do not appear to worry much and there is little social stress of the kind we undergo.

The dietary staple is "pinole" – corn that is parched and ground into a fine meal-like flour. This is mixed with water and usually made into a type of tortilla. The indians also eat beans that resemble brown beans, as well as fruit and berries off the land. They eat fish, too.

They have dignity, respect for law and other, high standards of behaviour, and do not lie or steal. Violence among them is rare and they treat opponents (in races) with courtesy and respect.'

Mr. Zahn asks, 'Can such people be called uncivilised?'

Whatever genetic or other factors may be postulated, could these Indians, who are 'generally as unhealthy as any other uncivilised people', manifest this activity at an altitude of 8,000 ft. if their nutrition was at fault?

Recent figures published by the Office of Health Economics, show that in 1966-1967, 301-million working days were lost in this country through certified sickness, at a cost of at least £1,200,000,000 a year. As *The Times* comments, this £1,200,000,000 estimate of lost production, does not include a large amount of unrecorded sickness absence. Add to this figure, the £261.8-million paid out by the Exchequer in sickness benefit and the £2,000,000,000 a year which the National Health Service is costing the taxpayers, together with the considerable cost of drugs bought privately, a round figure of £4,000,000,000 a year, due directly or indirectly to ill-health, is probably exceeded. *The Times* notes that figures show that the biggest single cause of absence from work continued to be bronchitis, which accounted for 12% of days lost, but the relatively minor illnesses, such as nervousness, debility and headache, had contributed substantially to the increase in absence over the past years and suggests that people are no longer prepared to ignore minor illnesses.

A recent random survey in London, of 1,000 people, aged 16 to 60, with detailed chemical blood and urine and chest x-ray examinations, showed that nine out of ten were, unfit. Of these, more than half were under 40. Apart from those who were already under medical attention, 519 were considered to have disabilities sufficient for them to be referred to their own doctors. Only 67 out of the 1,000 examined, were classed as completely fit.

As far as mortality figures are concerned, the O.H.E. publication, *The Age of Maturity,* gives some very depressing figures. This report emphasises that the over 45s had not benefitted from medical progress to anything like the same extent as the younger age group. The spectacular reduction in deaths from T.B. and infectious diseases has been offset by increase in lung cancer and heart disease. In this country alone, someone dies every ten minutes from cancer of the lung due to cigarette smoking. The then Minister of State for Health, Mr. David Ennals, when asked about lung cancer, said, 'We could save more lives by persuading people to stop smoking than by any other step I can think of. The big problem is indifference. Cigarette smokers think that smoking may be bad for other people but not for themselves, or they take the attitude, "I am prepared to risk it". Evidence is overwhelming from studies here and abroad, about the cancer link.' I mention this, not in any way to put you off smoking cigarettes, though you may prefer to avoid manslaughter through offering them to others, but to show how difficult it is to influence behaviour by telling an unpleasant truth. Nowadays, people hope to be absolved from paying the penalty of violating the laws of health, by taking a pill or by spare-part surgery. The lung cancer rate is rising in all sections of the community except one, namely, doctors, among whom there is a 30% drop. However, women at least are now beginning to regard smoking seriously. A new and appalling smoking hazard has recently come to light – facial wrinkles. I quote the *Medical Tribune* of 20th March: 'London: A doctor's observation has revealed a new smoking hazard and it has an electric effect on getting his women patients to give up cigarettes, namely, the finding that habitual smoking causes wrinkles.' Several doubting colleagues did their own studies and confirmed the doctor's findings. As to the effect on women, Dr. Daniels writes, 'Heart to heart talks and threats of catastrophic disease had but little effect compared to the diagnosis of impending 'crow's foot'.'

I have talked about smoking because it exemplifies what I believe to be a common cause of cancer, namely a local irritant acting on tissues whose nutrition has been impaired either by the irritant itself or for some other reason. Inhalation of a carcinogenic substance will naturally affect, first, the mouth, tongue, jaws, larynx, trachea and lungs, with a maximum incidence on the latter; then, through the presence of toxic substances in the swallowed saliva, is likely to affect the oesophagus and stomach and finally, after absorption and concentration in the urinary tract, produce growths in the bladder.

Food Additives: The number of food additives is now legion. Many of them are regarded as capable of producing cancer. A year or so ago doctors were flooded with advertisements and samples, recommending cyclamates to replace sugar. This coal-tar derivative, which has no food value whatever, is ten times sweeter than sugar and, to quote an advertising blurb, 'is ideal to use on cereals and fruit and in tea, coffee, etc. and in general cooking.' This stuff was then passed by the Ministry of Agriculture, which is also the Ministry of Food, as fit for human consumption. What do we know about its effect on the body? It has been shown that in some people, cyclamates break down to cyclohexylamine, causing significant breaks in the chromosomes: in other words, altering the very structure of our body cells in a way closely allied to the changes occurring in cancer. It is known in some cases to have caused liver damage and skin eruptions and gastro-enteritis in children. Authority in a 101 page report, has recommended, 'It would be prudent to adhere to an intake of 50mg per kilogram body weight per day.' What nonsense for an alleged food! This intake could easily be exceeded by a child taking fruit drinks containing a 'Ministry approved sweetener', The word 'cyclamate' does not appear on the label. The latest report on cyclamates has shown that, 'The ingestion of even a small amount of cyclamate, used in the form of a diet drink, has been found to block the action of antibiotics, the effect of which is reduced to one-quarter of what it should be'. (In other words, life-saving anti-biotics can be made totally ineffective by small doses of cyclamate.) Why are cyclamates used at all? Paradoxically, because they have no food value: that is to say, their calorific value is negligible. For this reason, they are recommended to replace sugar for slimming purposes. Even in this they fail. Dutch scientists have found 'that rats fed on cyclamates actually gained weight faster than rats fed on normal diet, apparently by artificially stimulating appetite and raising the efficiency with which they use their food.' In agriculture, this would, I believe, be termed a better conversion factor. It looks as though the chemists backed the wrong horse and that a better market would lie with pigs rather than men. So, why were cyclamates commended for health and beauty? The answer, as always, is economic. Or, shall we call it a specious rationalisation motivated by greed. Cyclamates are five times cheaper to produce than sugar.

This indictment of cyclamates has been validated by withdrawal from the market, ostensibly for further testing. The reason given was experimental evidence that cyclamates in very large dosage can cause bladder tumours in rats. But the real point is that it is a non-food and that at the time of its official approval as a food substitute, sufficient was known or suspected of its potential toxicity for a proviso by the advisory Scientific Committee concerned that it should be used in restricted quantities: a restriction inexcusable in a 'food stuff' and quite impracticable of fulfilment.

All chemical food additives are suspect and should be permitted only if it can be shown absolutely that they have no possible harmful, short-term or long-term effects either in themselves, or in their possible breakdown products, or by reacting with other ingested chemicals.

The only safe food is whole food in variety, with a good proportion of fresh fruit and saladings and a minimum of denatured carbohydrates.

I would like to define food, or diet, as covering what we habitually, or commonly and voluntarily, ingest. This will allow me to comment on two particular hazards. Tranquillisers and so-called stimulants of the central nervous system comprise 15% of all medical prescriptions. They cost this country about £23-million a year. Can it be supposed that these drugs, any more than alcohol though to a lesser degree, can be exempted from blame in contributing to the rising tide of accidents, which are the third largest cause of death in this country and estimated to cost about £1,000-million a year?

I mention antibiotics and would like to take a look at their use in animal farming. A very high proportion of animal food concentrates are laced with antibiotics and the agricultural market for these is lucrative to the extent of £20-million a year. Antibiotics are given to unnaturally increase weight. This does not, of course, result in any increase in nutritional value of the carcases. They are also given to suppress evidence of disease, in chicken, cattle, pigs and sheep, reared in the revolting conditions of a factory farm. As a result of this, germs are arising, producing diseases in man which are resistant to antibiotic therapy. Of these disease-producing germs, originating in the bowel, the most important is the Salmonella group, organisms which are closely allied to the typhoid bacilli. Movement of factory-farmed bull calves from the West Country to the growing areas of the North and East, has already resulted in several outbreaks of severe dysentery from salmonella infection. Chicken, roast on a rotary spit, are often unsufficiently cooked on the inside to kill the germs of salmonella.

The hazard to health through the misuse of antibiotics, has been increased by a recently discovered phenomenon known as resistance transfer. Harmless organisms, in the bowel for instance, may acquire resistance to antibiotics. This resistance they are able to pass on to organisms not previously exposed to antibiotics. Dr. E.S. Anderson, at the Enteric Reference Laboratory, Colindale, who is the acknowledged expert on enteric infection in this country, has expressed serious concern at the rise in incidence of resistant strains of salmonella organisms. As a result of the mass medication of calves by antibiotics by farmers, Dr. Anderson says that the human population is being exposed to a great risk of salmonella infection, and to the risk of the transfer of infective drug resistance to essentially human organism pathogens. Death in calves, due to salmonella infection, has increased ten-fold in the last ten years and, incidentally, a further 10 to 15% die from what is grandiloquently called the disadaptation syndrome. This means from the unhygienic conditions and harsh treatment associated with factory farming. A recent editorial on this subject in the *New England Journal of Medicine* concluded, 'Unless drastic measures are taken, physicians may find themselves back in the pre-antibiotic Middle Ages in the treatment of infectious diseases. The Swann Report on antibiotics has now condemned the use of some of them as a growth stimulant. The real answer is to improve the conditions of the animals so antibiotics are no longer a substitute for good husbandry.'

The second specific hazard that I want to deal with is the Pill. It is estimated that the contraceptive pill at any given time is now being taken by 20% of women of child-bearing age in the Western World. As a writer in *World Medicine* has recently pointed out, before long a vast majority of western women will have taken the Pill at some time in their lives. Those who take it have a four-fold risk of developing fatal thrombosis. They have an increased risk of developing cancer of the womb. Recently, a further risk has become apparent, namely, interference with the enzyme systems in the body, leading to exacerbation of potentially fatal disorders, such as disseminated lupus erythematosis, and to a functional deficiency of Pyridoxine, a member of the all important B group of vitamins, which comprises also Niaein, Folic Acid and Vitamin B12. Lack of Vitamin B6 can lead to convulsions. mental retardation, anaemia and bladder cancer, and toxaemia of pregnancy. The principal source in our diet is whole wheat, and 84% of Pyridoxine is milled out in 70% extraction flour. The relationship of the Pill to Pyridoxine deficiency, together with certain other significant metabolic aberrations, came under investigation when an increasing number of women on the Pill began to show signs of severe mental depression. Can, or will, the Pill be a factor in the rising rate of suicide? We simply do not know. The Pill has only been in use for about a decade and, as in smoking and the saccharine disease, it may well take twenty years or more before the long-term effects of the Pill are known. It is quite possible, as a writer in *World Medicine* pointed out recently, that we may be heading for personal and genetic disaster. It is true that the Pill has now been modified to meet some of these criticisms. But it still remains a health hazard.

Among the elderly, a recent study has shown widespread malnutrition to a previously unsuspected degree. A random sample of the six and a half million elderly people in this country, in an investigation sponsored by the Ministry of Health and recognised as representative of the whole, shows that four elderly people out of five are suffering from vitamin deficiency to a clinically significant degree, especially of the all-important B group of vitamins and frequently, also, of vitamin C, ascorbic acid. These deficiencies and the results of appropriate treatment have been well shown by Dr. Geoffrey Taylor, who has also recently shown that there is an enormously high rate of fungal infection of the mouth and tongue in the elderly, and has rightly suggested that it is unlikely that this infection is confined to the mouth. What the full significance of this infection is we do not know, but the extent of our knowledge of vitamins and nutrition is eclipsed by the extent of our ignorance. A leading article in the *British Medical Journal*, dated 13th September 1969 and headed 'Old Age, Nutrition and Mental Confusion', points out that the increasing number of elderly people admitted to mental hospitals has shown mental illness which is frequently the result of dietetic deficiency. These may result in the sequence of faecal impaction, distension of the bladder, urinary infection, mental confusion and, finally, death; or diabetes which must be regarded as another nutritional disorder, or through lack of vitamin B12, which gives rise to severe psychiatric symptoms, or to deficiency of folic acid, leading to dementia. This end result of often life-long disordered nutrition is, I am sure you will agree, an appalling reflection on our mode of living.

Finally, I come to what is probably the greatest dietetic hazard of all, namely, refined carbohydrates.

In England, around a hundred years ago, two profound changes occurred in our eating habits. Roller-ground bleached flour began to replace whole-meal flour, and the chemically doctored white loaf, deficient in salts, vitamins and bran, became our stable fare. At about the same time, there was an enormous increase in consumption of the main source of carbohydrates, namely, refined sugar. Consumption of sugar has risen 800% and now averages over one cwt. per annum for every man, woman and child, as against 15lb. per annum in the first half of the nineteenth century.

The 70% extraction white loaf, as we know it today, was reintroduced in 1956 – not as alleged, at the request of the public who have come to loathe it, the public were in fact never asked – but like cyclamates, as a commercial proposition. In the discarded 30% fraction, which is sold as offal for pigs, and also back to us expensively as a wheat-germ supplement, goes all the germ containing the most valuable part of the protein and the vitamins and the bran, which prevents bowel stasis with all its attendant ills. It is then by law 'fortified' by chalk and by iron in an almost certainly useless form, and by a moiety of synthetic vitamin B1. The white loaf is a political confidence trick of no mean order!

Three years ago, I was working for four months in Sierra Leone as a surgeon in a Bush Hospital, among Africans living tribally. Infectious diseases take a heavy toll. In areas remote from medical care, four children out of five die before their fifth birthday. Anaemia, malaria, typhoid and tuberculosis, leprosy and bilharziasis are rife. But, and this is the most important point, the degenerative diseases which bedevil the western world are almost entirely non-existent. As a generalisation the ailments from which primitive people suffer are those which we have the knowledge to

131

cure, whereas we suffer from degenerative diseases of our own devising, which we cannot cure and have not yet learnt to prevent. These include coronary arterial disease and varicose veins, dental caries and diabetes, and many diseases of the gastro-intestinal tract and its associated glands. In this category are peptic ulcer, appendicitis and gall-bladder diseases, all of which have shown a phenomenal increase in this century, and others now common, crippling and often lethal, such as Crohn's disease or regional ileitis and ulcerative colitis, as well as diverticulitis of the colon, which have only appeared as clinical entities in the last sixty years.

The *World Tribune* of 29th August, 1969, under the heading 'Rise in Enteric Ills, reflects disturbed Ecology', reports the views of one of the world's leading enterologists. Dr. B.B. Crohn, Professor of Medicine at Mount Sinai Hospital, New York, draws attention to the vast amount of invalidism from ulcerative and degenerative conditions of the bowel, conditions which were not recognised sixty years ago and which, as Dr. Crohn states, 'could not have eluded the exquisitely accurate studies of great medical scientists at the turn of the century.' If those diseases did not exist, he declares, then they are new diseases. They cannot be attributed to the stresses of the 20th Century. Other centuries have also been marked by stress. Is the causation, he continues, to be found in the food we eat? What, he asks, is in the diet of Europeans that is different from the rice or native diet of the plurality of natives? Dr. Crohn concludes, 'Since these diseases fall into none of the categories of bacterial or viral aetiology, let us look further afield for the rapid evolution and spread. Let us look into the disturbed ecology of the human race.'

You will naturally ask, could they have been overlooked or given a different name? The accurate and detailed description of morbid anatomists and clinicians of the last century, rules out this suggestion.

The one and only major change in our dietetic habits lies in the refinement and concentration of carbohydrates. The strongest possible evidence incriminating this change as the cause of the degenerative diseases of the western world is given by Surgeon-Captain Cleave and his Associates, in their book entitled, *Diabetes, Coronary Thrombosis and the Saccharine Disease,* as you can read in Captain Cleave's article in this book. From this, the conclusion can only be drawn that return to wholefood would immeasurably reduce the appalling load of ill-health in this country and effect a tax saving to be reckoned probably in hundreds of millions of pounds.

These, then, are our troubles. They are not to be put right by bread alone, not even whole wheat bread. We have got to discover, or re-discover, the laws of the universe and to obey them. We need a new attitude of mind, a new quality of life. We have become bemused by technological achievements. Scientific idolatry is linked with cosmic impiety. There is a historic coincidence between the growing disbelief in God and the increasing propensity to abuse and despoil nature, even human nature. Through greed and selfishness and materialism, which is the father of all 'isms', we have exploited our heritage. The Astronomer Royal, Jeans, said, 'The Universe begins to look more like a great thought than like a great machine. We discover the Universe shows signs of the designing or controlling power that has something in common with our own individual mind.'

The more we discover of the Universe and its workings, the more we discover of God and his workings. Thy will be done on earth states a fundamental law for healthy living.

9. Poisons in our food

Dr. Kenneth Mellanby

Dr. Mellanby who has held many distinguished posts in education and research is now Director of the Nature Conservancy's Experimental Station at Monks Wood, Huntingdon. He is also Chairman of the Soil Association's Research Advisory Committee.

IT IS FIRST necessary to consider briefly the subject of toxicology. Poisons are substances which are defined as being harmful to living organisms. However, the nature of this harm, and the amount of a poisonous substance which can cause harm, differs enormously. There are, for instance, toxins produced by some micro-organisms which are so poisonous that if a small fraction of a milligram enters the human body, death immediately occurs. At the other end of the scale, almost anything can be defined as a poison if too much is taken, or if it is taken in the wrong way. This means that we have to have some sort of scale of toxicity.

Then poisons can be divided into two classes, acute poisons and chronic poisons. Cyanide is an example of an acute poison – if you take a single large enough dose, you die. But if you take only a tiny amount, no damage is done. Furthermore, you may repeat these tiny doses day after day, and there is still no noticeable effect, for the cyanide is rapidly broken down into harmless products. Aspirin again, though far less toxic, can also be an acute poison; many people have committed suicide by taking one massive dose of about an ounce (200 tablets). But many other people take several milligrams of aspirin every day of their lives without appearing to come to any harm. Now, as regards acute toxicity, aspirin is just about as poisonous as is the insecticide DDT. About one ounce of DDT is, for man, a lethal dose. But if we take, every day, the same sort of amount of DDT as people do of aspirin, the result is quite different. The DDT is, for the most part, retained within the body; it is not broken down or excreted as is the aspirin. Thus if a man ingests a hundredth of an ounce of DDT a day, he will eventually build up a toxic amount in his body. This will not happen in a hundred days, for some of the DDT is lost, but probably the build-up will occur within 200 days. The same thing can happen with some chronic poisons in food.

There is another quite different, but equally dangerous, chronic effect caused particularly by some additives to sophisticated foods, but which can also occur from the ingestion of naturally-occurring substances. This is most easily demonstrated in the case of carcinogens – substances which, perhaps taken in minute amounts over a long period, produce some form of cancer. Here the continued exposure to a low concentration is the damage; there need be no build-up of the chemical.

Finally there are the apparently non-poisonous substances which are dangerous when present in the wrong amounts or in the wrong places. It has often been said that even common salt in large enough doses is a poison. Other dangers arise from the way in which food crops are grown. All plants contain nitrates, and trace elements which are essential for growth of plants and animals, but if nitrates or trace elements are present in too high concentrations, toxic effects may result. Vitamins are clearly necessary for health, but even vitamins are dangerous if taken in excessive amounts. The most obvious case is vitamin A. Vitamin A is essential for human health, but dangerous amounts can be taken in overdoses of pharmaceutical preparations, and even by over-indulging in natural foods. The classic case of illness from excessive intake of vitamin A is in shipwrecked sailors who have eaten the liver of polar bears. Polar bear liver contains, naturally, a very high concentration of

K

vitamin A, built up by concentrating the vitamin A in the animals which form the bear's diet.

When we consider the effects of poisons, we often speak of the LD_{50}. This is easily determined when an insecticide is used on a population of pest insects. In a series of experiments the dose of the insecticide is increased. A low dose gives a negligible effect, but as the dose is increased so the number of deaths increases. The LD_{50} is the dose which kills half the insects. The LD_{50} of most poisons for man cannot be so accurately assessed, but, as the result of accidents and by extrapolation from animal experiments, some reasonable estimate can be made. As a general rule it is then assumed that a dose of an acute poison less than a fiftieth of the LD_{50} can be tolerated; experience shows that, in most cases, this assumption is justified, and that this margin of safety is a reasonable one. We observe this sort of standard when we are concerned with poisonous substances which may get into our food. But there are many natural foods which contain poisons in quantities far higher than the LD_{50}. Were these synthetic substances, they would immediately be banned from our diet. Perhaps we are too lax in our regulations regarding natural foods.

Potatoes are a case in point. These vegetables normally contain some 90 parts per million of poisonous solanine; this is only about a fifth (not a fiftieth, the level often accepted for synthetic foods) of the dangerous level, and potatoes which have been exposed to light do in fact easily reach this danger level. Then both spinach and rhubarb contain oxalate in amounts which could be harmful to the greedy eater. Oxalate levels in rhubarb stalks are high enough for safety, but the leaves are much more poisonous, and numerous deaths have occurred, particularly in wartime, when these leaves have been cooked as a substitute for spinach. As mentioned above, oxalate levels in spinach itself are considerable, and I often think that the natural reaction of many babies, who actively eject spinach forced on them in the mistaken idea that it will do them good, may be instinctively correct. Serious poisoning has also resulted from over-indulgence in such things as avocados, onions and horseradish – horseradish contains substantial amounts of mustard oil, and has killed pigs, horses and cattle though, so far, no human deaths have been reported.

These vegetables are usually poisonous only if eaten in abnormally large amounts. Other foods need special treatment if they are to be reasonably safe. Thus cassava, which is one of the staple carbohydrate foods of the tropics, contains large amounts of cyanide. If cassava is eaten without previous fermentation, lethal amounts of cyanide can easily be taken. The amount of cyanide in almonds and cherry stones is also appreciable, but these seldom form a large enough part of anyone's diet to be harmful, though I remember a detective story where there was sufficient poison in the first glass poured from the top of a bottle of cherry brandy to claim a victim. However, I do not think that death from this cause is very likely in practice.

The poisons so far considered have been taken unintentionally. We also deliberately take other poisonous substances. One of these is alcohol, which most of us think of as a pleasant vice, as indeed it is in moderation. However, alcohol is in fact an acute poison, and were it invented today by some chemical firm, it would not have the slightest chance of being permitted as an article for human consumption. We do, at the moment, have at least 300,000 people in Britain seriously ill from alcohol poisoning, and many others who are intermittently poisoned and whose health and efficiency is affected. Caffein, the active principle in tea and coffee, is also a poison, and chronic tea and coffee drinkers do suffer from toxic effects. Custom and time make us accept many substances which would otherwise be condemned. I personally list 'wine' as one of my hobbies in *Who's Who,* and I am an inveterate tea and coffee drinker.

The toxicity of foods may be modified by the way in which they are grown. Increased bulk of most vegetable crops may be produced by giving heavy dressings of inorganic nitrates to the soil. Many of us consider that the

result is food of inferior quality and taste, but it can sometimes also be dangerous. Some vegetables, particularly our
old friend spinach, take up nitrates in such large amounts
as to render the crop dangerous (quite apart from·its oxalate
content) to babies. Considerable amounts of canned
vegetable baby foods have been condemned as poisonous
in the United States because of their high nitrate content.
Adults could probably consume these *purées* without harm
(if with little enjoyment) but the flora of the gut in infants
is different, nitrates may be broken down to nitrites, and
this combines with the haemoglobin in the blood to form
met- haemoglobin which does not carry oxygen and the
victim may be literally asphyxiated. Vegetables grown
organically will not contain these high nitrate levels –
though even organic spinach has sufficient oxalate to make
it suspect as an infant food.

So far we have dealt with natural poisons; civilised man
also deliberately adds toxic substances to sophisticated
foods, to 'improve' their appearance, their taste or their
keeping power. We have a complicated machinery for
testing these additives, and I think that there is no doubt
that the majority are harmless. They are certainly less
dangerous than some of the naturally-occurring poisons we
have been discussing. However, accidents do happen, preliminary tests do not always exclude chemicals later found
to be harmful, and I think we are right to be suspicious of
these additives. We now ban cyclamates as sweeteners,
though in this case many scientists think that they are less
dangerous than the sugar they replace. Butter yellow
(p-dimethylaminoazobenzene) was used as a food colour
for many years before it was shown to cause cancer in rats.
Agene (the gas nitrogen trichloride) was used to improve
flour, and only discontinued when it was realised that it
had toxic effects, recognised by the hysteria it induced in
dogs. It is a comment on our civilisation that with one
hand we remove the flavour and the nutrients from our
food, and then we put back what is often the wrong taste
and the wrong chemical. Our instinct for pure, whole food

is undoubtedly right, but difficult to indulge by all the millions crowded into our cities.

Otherwise-wholesome foods may be accidentally made poisonous. A classic case is that of groundnuts, used in animal foods and for making margarine. Some ten years ago outbreaks of what was at first thought of as a new disease occurred in turkeys and other birds; deaths also occurred in laboratory animals. Finally the cause was found to be a poison called aflatoxin, produced by a fungus which infested groundnuts stored under warm and humid conditions. This is in fact a particular case of 'food poisoning'; it occurred in food not originally thought of as perishable. We are all familiar with the danger from meat, fish, etc., kept too long under warm conditions.

Radiation may also endanger our food. The testing of atomic weapons has raised the level of radiation in a number of foods, including milk. So far the level is low, and the exposure to any individual is only a small fraction of the normal background radiation inevitably experienced. However, after an accident at the Windscale Power Station, large supplies of milk from farms in the vicinity were destroyed because the level of radiation in it was considered unacceptable. The disposal of radio-active waste from nuclear power stations is an increasingly serious problem, and one which could give world-wide danger. At present the level of waste emission from power stations in Britain is restricted severly, so that even seaweeds and lobsters, which concentrate radio-active elements from the sea, offer no danger even to those most addicted to these forms of food. At present we have been reasonably responsible regarding industrial radiation, and military testing has been at least reduced by the more responsible countries, but in the long term radiation as a form of food poisoning could be very serious.

Finally we come to pesticides, poisonous substances used to kill organisms considered detrimental by man. We use herbicides to poison weeds, fungicides to poison fungi and insecticides to poison insects. All these substances are poisonous to man and to animals as well as to the plants or insects against which they are directed, but nevertheless chemists have succeeded in producing pesticides with considerable selectivity, which thus kill the target pest at doses which appear to do little harm to other forms of life. When carefully used, many modern pesticides do the maximum good in controlling pests and have the minimum of harmful side effects. Nevertheless there is always some danger, and the search for successful non-chemical methods of pest control is one which we would all wish to encourage.

Fortunately the most acutely toxic pesticides are less commonly used today. Herbicides like DNOC and insecticides like parathion were the cause of fatal accidents to man and animals. Parathion was a common suicide drug. Food treated with these chemicals was dangerously toxic, but only for a short time after they were applied. The ecological advantage of these very poisonous pesticides was that they were not persistent, and broke down to comparatively harmless residues in hours or, at most, days. Thus they did not have such serious long-term effects as other, apparently less dangerous, chemicals, which were more persistent.

Few of the herbicides, or of the organophosphorus insecticides, in wide use in Britain today, seem to be a serious cause of food contamination. They have important and sometimes unfortunate ecological effects, particularly when improperly used, but their long-term dangers seem to be minimal. The chemicals which cause most concern are the organochlorine insecticides, including DDT, dieldrin, heptachlor and endosulfan. The reason for their danger lies in their chemical properties. They are persistent, not easily broken down either in the soil or in living organisms – they are not easily 'biodegradable'. Some chemical changes, particularly in living tissues, do take place, but the products of these reactions are still very insecticidal, sometimes in fact more strongly insecticidal than their precursors. The other important property of the organochlorine insecticides is that though they are only very sparingly soluble in water, they are very soluble in fat. This enables animals to extract these chemicals from very low concentrations in water or in foods, and to store them in their body tissues.

In 1967 the average Briton had about 3 parts per million of organochlorine insecticide, mainly DDT and its metabolites, in his body. This represented a level of between ten and fifty times that found in most common foods, so a considerable degree of concentration had taken place. It is interesting to note, however, that this body level had remained fairly constant for some ten years. There has been a balance between intake and excretion (and breakdown) of the insecticides. In the United States, levels of insecticides in tissues are about 12 parts per million, much higher than in Britain, but here again these tissue levels have kept fairly steady for several years. The indication is that today these tissue levels are beginning to fall. There is still some insecticide in the food, but it is decreasing and the level of tissue concentration is falling also. This equilibrium is important; we should realise that *all* the insecticide ingested is not retained, and that the tissue level bears some relation to the level in the food.

The important question is: what do these tissue levels signify? Are we in any way endangered by having these amounts of insecticides in our tissues? It seems probable that we are not. The reason for this assumption is that many people have had far higher levels for many years without showing any harmful symptoms. Workers in factories formulating insecticidal preparations get much more heavily contaminated. Eventually the insecticides can rise to levels where they have pathological effects, but there is no evidence that fat levels of even 100 parts per million in man (i.e. at least 30 times higher than is commonly found in Britain) are harmful. There seems a reasonable margin of safety. Nevertheless it is dangerous to be dogmatic, and scientists agree on the desirability of reducing or even eliminating this contamination of human tissues. But in general it is safe to say that, so far, DDT levels contaminating our food have not had seriously harmful effects.

When we consider the harmful ecological effects that organochlorine insecticides have had on wildlife, particularly in America, but also to some extent in Britain, this statement may be surprising. However, it must be realised that wildlife particularly in fresh water, has suffered a quite different degree of exposure. Recognition of this has resulted in drastic restrictions on the use of these insecticides, and these have taken effect in most cases before man has been seriously affected.

We see that our food presents many dangers. It contains poisons from natural sources, and poisons that are present because of human activities. Nevertheless, though these substances can endanger health, I do not think that they are generally such a danger as an unbalanced diet of sophisticated, but nutritionally impoverished foods. The efforts of the Soil Association to encourage the production of pure, unadulterated and natural food are steps in the right direction, but even these desirable foods must be combined in the proper ratios, and too great quantities of even those natural foods with high levels of toxic substances are probably better avoided.

10. Changing patterns of disease

A. Elliot-Smith, F.R.C.S., formerly Senior Surgeon, Radcliffe Infirmary, Oxford

Mr. Elliot-Smith has always been convinced of the recent appearance of many of our present day diseases: he proved it to his own satisfaction by going through the records of his hospital. Service in the Middle East during the war and work in Libya since retirement has strengthened his convictions.

TOWARDS the end of the 19th century it became apparent that the pattern of disease was changing. Previously rare diseases were becoming much more common and new diseases were being recognised. When a new disease is announced it is often suggested that this is an old disease newly recognised, and that the bedside clinician of a hundred years ago was often unable correctly to diagnose the malady. There may be some truth in this contention, but at least the pathologist carrying out the examination after death was usually able to say what had been the cause of death, although, as we shall later see, even the postmortem findings are capable of misinterpretation.

It is established, therefore, that about the turn of the century new diseases did begin to appear.

An experience whilst dealing with surgical outpatients in August 1967 may emphasise some of the changes that have occurred. Amongst many patients seen that day four remain in my memory: a case of duodenal ulcer, afflicting a young man with crippling attacks of recurrent pain; a case of gallstones; another of rather severe varicose veins, and finally a case of chronic appendicitis. It may be fairly said that these

143

are the usual types of case seen in surgical outpatients every day all over the country; nothing exceptional about them. But there are two points of interest and importance: all four patients were in their teens. and when the young of our nation suffer crippling disease it behoves the doctors to ask 'Why?'

The second point of interest is that all these four diseases can be considered twentieth century 'plagues'; they were all very rare or unknown a hundred years ago.

The Rise of Appendicitis

Appendicitis has always been a fascinating disease to surgeons, because there are not many conditions which will reduce a person from complete health and normality to a state nigh unto death within 48 hours of onset. A bad case of appendicitis will do this, and therefore correct diagnosis and early treatment are essential to avoid risk to life.

This disease was first described in England by a London surgeon, Vince Parkinson, in 1812. He described very accurately the illness and postmortem appearances of a boy of 5 who died after four days of a perforated appendix. Death was due to generalised peritonitis starting in the vicinity of the perforation.

Appendicitis therefore was not unknown in the 19th century but it was a very rare occurrence.

I have studied the annual reports of the last hundred years of the Radcliffe Infirmary, Oxford, with particular attention to the rise in incidence of appendicitis. The Radcliffe Infirmary celebrated its bicentenary last year (1970), having opened for the treatment of inpatients in October 1770, and it has been most interesting to see the pattern of work which has gone on in the hospital as it expanded from a mere 100 beds to the present 600.

When a new disease appears it is not always recognised for exactly what it is. Appendicitis was for a long time thought to start as inflammation of the caecum (the portion of the large bowel to which the appendix is

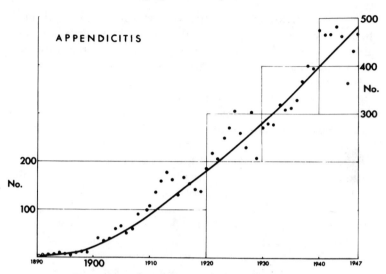

Fig. 1.—Cases of appendicitis at the Radcliffe Infirmary.

attached) and the condition was referred to as typhlitis, indicating inflammation of the typhlos or caecum. Later it was realised that the inflammation was around the caecum but not originating in the caecum: it was therefore referred to as perityphlitis. In 1895 the true origin of the disease was finally realised and the term appendicitis came into use. When studying hospital records and in view of these different terms, it is important to consider all cases of typhlitis, perityphlitis, caecal abscess, caecal fistula and appendicitis as examples of one disease. If this is done, in the Radcliffe records up to 1895 the annual total of these cases varies between 5 – 10 a year. After this date there has been a dramatic rise in the incidence, by 1905 there are 40 cases a year and by 1930, 300 annually, and at the present time there are over 500 cases each year.

Duodenal Ulcer

This is another disease which shows an increasing pattern; the Radcliffe Infirmary records mention it first in 1891.

We are fortunate in having very definite figures about peptic ulcer including duodenal ulcer as it occurred in the British Army. To have a proven ulcer, either gastric or duodenal, has always been grounds for discharge from the Army, and we therefore have some accurate figures for such discharges in two world wars.

From August 1914 until the end of 1915 there were 709 discharges on account of ulcer. From September 1939 until the end of 1941, a period of time approximately twice that of the first war, in which one might expect about twice the number of ulcer cases compared to 1914, there were in fact 23,500 men discharged with proven ulcers.

As can be imagined, these facts caused considerable concern in Army medical circles and an explanation was sought for the extraordinary increase in the occurrence of ulcer. It was first suggested that the Army cooks and Army food was the cause, and true enough in the first war any soldier too dim to hold a rifle was sent to the cook-house to peel potatoes; but in the second world war a new idea emerged, cooks were taught to cook, a Catering Corps was formed, efficient rationing was instituted at the outbreak of war and the Services had first call on food supplies. It was therefore unlikely that Army food was the explanation of ulcer.

The next suggestion was that it might be psychic trauma, separation of families, danger, etc. But in the opening phase of each war there were notable differences: in the first there was great slaughter from the beginning, many thousands of casualties in the first few months, whilst in the second war the first stage was called the 'phoney war'. We had an Expeditionary Force in France which marched and trained, dug trenches, had sing-songs and drank countless cups of NAAFI tea, but there was no fighting until the brief campaign which ended in Dunkirk. The theory of psychic trauma and danger did not explain the boat-loads of ulcer patients returning from France.

The next idea was to obtain a detailed history of the symptoms from a number of the soldiers returning sick.

It was found that in the great majority of patients their dyspepsia antedated their entrance into the Army by a number of years: they already had ulcers when they enlisted. The ulcer patient admissions to six hospitals were next investigated and it was found that between 1925 and 1929 there was a dramatic rise in the number of cases. This was a great puzzle, but it was the explanation why so many men in the Army had ulcers. During the late twenties was the time of the severe post-war depression. There was a crash on the New York Stock Exchange, there was depression and unemployment all over Europe and America. The unemployment rate in Britain exceeded two million and for the unemployed in those days the 'dole' was not very adequate. In fact starvation was not far distant and bread and margarine was far from an adequate diet. It is possible that this time of financial depression may have been in part responsible for the rise of ulcers in the late twenties, but if this is so it is difficult to explain the maintenance of the ulcer rate through the thirties when the depression had disappeared. An alternative factor may be that agene was introduced into British flour at this time. Agene we now know is a poisonous substance; it produces hysteria in dogs. This 'flour improver' has now been prohibited and has been replaced by other substances.

These are the facts related to the rise of appendicitis and duodenal ulcer; similar evidence can be produced to show the recent increase in many other diseases common in Britain today: coronary thrombosis, diabetes, ulcerative colitis, diverticulitis and even varicose veins.

Speculation

We shall now switch from facts to speculation as to why these diseases have occurred.

Asiatic people and Africans do not suffer from these new diseases that are so prevalent in Europe and America, provided they stay in their own countries and pursue their traditional way of life. But if they come to live in western countries they may soon fit in with the patterns of disease that prevail in their new land.

Referring again to evidence from the British Army which has always been composed of many nationalities, Sikhs, Gurkhas, Basutos, Sudanese and many others: when on active service many of these troops had their own native food, whilst others, for example the Sudanese, were very proud to have British Army rations. It was noticed by Army surgeons in the Middle East that many Sudanese came into hospital with surgical diseases similar to the U.K. troops, appendicitis, duodenal ulcer, etc., whilst the troops on their own native diet did not have these diseases at all. Here is a strong suggestion that food was the cause.

It has long been observed that the American Negroes suffer just as frequently from these new diseases as the white Americans, yet their genetic brothers in Africa do not suffer from them.

Diet

It seems, therefore, that these diseases may be due to changes in our diet. Various investigations have suggested that there is probably some alteration in the fat, especially animal fat, that is consumed nowadays. This is a difficult theory to accept. Animal fat in the diet has been blamed for a lot of present diseases, but it is an extraordinary thing that a substance which man has been consuming for thousands of years should suddenly in the 20th century become poisonous to him! Thus the theory about fat is not proven.

Protein consumption has not altered significantly; western countries always eat more protein as meat compared to eastern countries where the diet is mainly vegetable.

The Role of Sugar

The carbohydrate in our diet has shown considerable change in quantity and quality over the last 100 years.

Carbohydrate is of two distinct types: it can be either sugar, or starch which we get from cereals.

The consumption of refined sugar per head of the population has increased in the most remarkable way during the past century. In the middle of the 18th century we were consuming about 4 lb. per head per year, practically nothing; in 1850 we were consuming about 25 lb. per head per year and now the rate is about 125 lb. per head per year. This 125 lb. a year does not tell the whole story, for many people nowadays are aware that sugar should not be eaten in excessive amounts and curtail their consumption; there must therefore be others who consume two or three times the average quantity.

Sugar has been called 'empty calories' because it provides calories and nothing else, neither essential vitamins not protein, so that if an excess of sugar is eaten it follows that less carbohydrate is taken of a type which might be more beneficial.

If we now consider the other carbohydrate component of our diet, flour made from cereals, we find that about 1872 a profound change occurred which affected adversely the nutritive quality of flour. At this time the milling of wheat changed from stone grinding in a multitude of mills all over the country, to roller milling by steel rollers in fewer large mills mainly near the ports. The effect of this change was to remove from this flour most of the bran and wheat germ with their mineral and vitamin content, especially vitamins B and E.

These facts suggest that an excess of sugar together with the impoverished nutritional value of our flour may be the explanation of many of our present diseases.

This theory as it concerns sugar was enunciated in Britain (in detail) by Surgeon-Captain T.L. Cleave, R.N., in the *Journal of the Royal Navy Medical Service* in 1956 and further elaborated in his book, *Diabetes, Coronary Thrombosis and the Saccharine Disease,* 1966.

In conclusion it is reasonable to suggest that correction of dietetic faults by a reduction in sugar consumption together with a restoration of the nutritive value of our flour would lead to a diminishing toll of disease and an overall improvement in health.

11. Is there a correlation between the health of a population and the method of husbandry used to produce its food?

T.W. McSheehy, B.Sc., M.I.Biol., F.R.S.H., Head of Department of Nutrition, Soil Association Research Laboratories

The Soil Association Research Farms are divided into three sections, each one employing a different method of husbandry. McSheehy discusses how the products of different systems may affect the health of the consumer.

ANY attempt to answer this question without reference to the soil would be incomplete and here the term soil is used in its broadest sense to include the highly complex biological and chemical interactions that *in toto* form the complete soil ecosystem. A system which has evolved over a very long period of time and which has never become static.

The evolution of the British Isles took about 4,500 million years and for the greater part of this time they were situated near the centre of an enormous super-continent called Pangaea (Fig. 1). This land mass was always on the move and as time passed, geological time measured in millions of years, the surface was subjected to many different environments. At one stage a particular area may have been beneath a shallow sea; later this very same area may have been traversed by a range of mountains. Climatic conditions ranged from arctic cold to desert heat; from tropical rain to very dry. The overall effect of these diverse changes collectively known as weathering was the production of the soil essential for life on the land. Once the soil

L

151

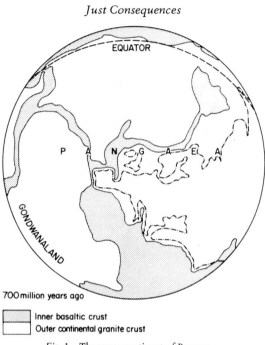

700 million years ago

Inner basaltic crust
Outer continental granite crust

Fig. 1.–The super-continent of Pangaea.

had been established there followed the evolution of plant and animal life. Starting with simple forms of living organisms the process gradually gathered momentum and the primitive soil ecosystem became increasingly more complex leading eventually to the production of a vast number of different species. The climax of this evolutionary process is found in those animals which have their own inbuilt mechanisms for maintaining homeostasis. In other words compensating control mechanisms which maintain the temperature, humidity, electrolyte balance, etc., of the body sensibly constant irrespective of external environment.

As the volume of plant and animal life increased so competition for an existence intensified. This factor, together with climatological changes, led to the extinction of many species. The vacant ecological niches so created were filled by the evolution of new species or by an existing species expanding its environmental boundaries.

Recently, in the last two million years, a new genus evolved. Although this produced several species only one, *Homo sapiens,* survived. This one species, however, was to exert more influence on the environment and hence on the ecosystem than had previously been possible by plants and animals and Man's impact on the ecology of the planet even now is not fully appreciated.

For a long time Man was a hunter and even in Neolithic times when the population of the British Isles was only 20,000, corn growing was still subsidiary to pasture farming. Gradually Man became less nomadic and his role within the ecosystem changed. Ploughing of the land with its concomitant change in the flora and fauna became the accepted practice of the day. During the early stages of the agricultural evolution the areas of land under cultivation were small and the repercussions within the ecosystem were insignificant. As agriculture developed and larger areas came under cultivation the ecological effects became progressively more important.

In his efforts to improve growing conditions for his crops Man created environments particularly suitable, or unsuitable, for a number of other plants and animals. An unfortunate corollary of planting a large area of wheat is the increase in the population of insects that feed on this plant. It is not very long before the insects are competing with Man for the produce and at this stage he has to instigate control measures. For many years rotation of crops proved to be reasonably effective and the long term ecological consequences were not disturbing. During the last fifty years, however, with the advent of chemical pesticides, herbicides, etc., the effects on the biosphere have become increasingly more noticeable (Fig. 2). Apart from their lack of specificity many of these compounds have very long half-lives and it is well known that some organochlorine insecticides, such as DDT and dieldrin, are universally present in fresh water and marine ecosystems[1]. Even Antarctic penguins have DDT in their body fat deposits.

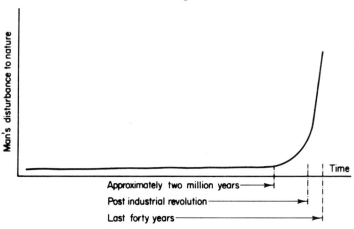

Fig. 2.—Man's disturbance to Nature.

Another important though less dramatic change in the soil ecosystem is being produced by modern farming techniques which have substituted pure chemical fertilisers for the impure heterogenous mixture of chemicals known as farm-yard manure. It is generally accepted that there are thirteen elements essential for normal plant growth and development but fertiliser applications are still restricted to three or four elements. The thirteen elements interact with one another and it is not possible to alter the concentration of one element within the soil without influencing the availability of others. An oversimplification of these processes is depicted by Mulder[2] in his interaction chart (Fig. 3). Since there are variations in the mineral requirements of different species this chart can only be taken as a general indication of the situation found in many plants. It can be seen, for example, that a high concentration of soil phosphorus will antagonise the uptake of copper, zinc and potassium. Low phosphate level is the growth limiting factor in many soils and their fertility can be increased by applications of phosphatic fertilisers. Unfortunately there is always the temptation to overdose the land and there is abundant evidence that this can lead to zinc deficiency in

154

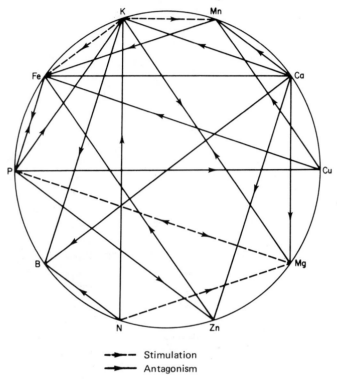

━▶━ ─ Stimulation
━▶━━ Antagonism

Fig. 3.—Mulder's interaction chart.

the crops[3-8]. This, however, is only part of the overall effect since heavy applications of phosphate can also significantly increase the molybdenum content of the herbage[9] and this can lead to copper deficiency in cattle grazing on the pasture.

There are many examples of an association between soil conditions and animal health and there is some evidence that these factors may also play a part in human disease. Ludwig *et al*[10] consider that in parts of New Zealand the incidence of dental caries is positively correlated with low molybdenum levels in the soil. These observations supported earlier findings by Ter Meulen[11], Adler and Straul[12], and Nagy and Polyik[13]. Legon[14] presents evidence of an association between abdominal cancer and soil type and Griffith[15] discusses the possibilities at greater length in his *Soil and Cancer*.

There is no doubt that soil conditions can influence the health of animals including Man and in part the question posed by the title of this paper has been answered. If, however, one enquires further and asks whether there is a difference in the nutritional quality of food produced by orthodox farming techniques, which use artificial fertilisers and biologically active sprays, and those methods which use mainly farm-yard manure, composts, and no chemical sprays the answer becomes largely hypothetical. At the present time very little information is available on the relative nutritional value of, for example, wheat grown by these two methods of farming.

To evaluate the question it is important to consider in greater detail the relationship between the soil and the plant, or more specifically between the environment and that part of the plant which is particularly concerned with absorption. This process occurs to some extent over most of the plant, hence the success of systemic herbicides, but there is a specialised part of the root system, called the piliferous layer or root-hair region, which is specifically designed as an absorption area. The cells of this region have a characteristic shape which greatly increases the ratio of surface area to cell volume (Fig. 4). These root-hairs are relatively small structures varying in diameter from 5 – 17 microns and 80 – 1500 microns in length[16]. In the young root-hair the cellulose cell wall is covered externally with a plastic layer of pectic acid but as the cell matures this mucilaginous layer is converted into a hard skin of calcium pectate. Once this has happened the cell is no longer concerned with absorption. Between the cell wall and the cytoplasm that lines it there is an interfacial membrane called the plasma membrane. This is a differentiated highly organised part of the cytoplasm particularly concerned with the passage of ions and nutrients into and out of the cell. The structure of cell membranes is remarkably con-

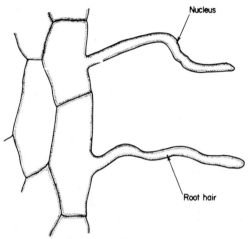

Fig. 4.–Root hairs.

stant for all living cells, irrespective of whether they are from plant or animal species. They all contain about 60% protein and 40% lipids, most of which are in the form of phospholipids. They all have a high electrical resistance and a low surface tension and their molecular organisation appears to be very similar in that they consist basically of a sandwich of lipids between two layers of protein. The phospholipid molecules are polarised with their hydrophilic parts outermost and their hydrophobic hydrocarbon chains innermost (Fig. 5).

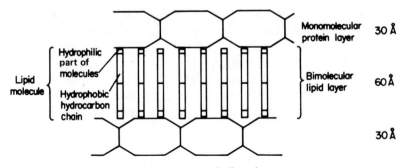

Fig. 5. -Structure of cell membrane.

157

These membranes vary in their permeability to different solutes. Some solute molecules, particularly those that have no electrical charge, are able to pass through the membrane by simple diffusion. In the majority of cases the rate at which they do this is directly proportional to their solubility in oil. One notable exception is water which in spite of a low solubility in oil passes through membranes very readily. Charged ions such as K^+ and Na^+ do not pass through membranes as easily. There are no large 'holes' in the surface of the membrane through which the solute molecules can pass. They cross by first dissolving in one side of the membrane then diffusing through the middle lipid layer and finally dissolving out the other side. The driving force is provided by the inherent tendency of the solute molecules to randomise themselves throughout the membrane – the so called 'diffusion force'. This process ceases when the concentration of solute has equilibrated across the membrane.

The solute composition on one side of a cell membrane may be very different from that on the other side. This difference may be maintained throughout the life of the cell in spite of the membrane being permeable to the solutes in question. A consideration of the intracellular and extracellular levels of sodium ions (Na^+) and potassium ions (K^+) in the red blood cells illustrates this point. Sodium ions inside the erythrocyte are maintained at a concentration of about five millimolar (mM) compared with an outside blood plasma concentration of about 150mM. The opposite is true for potassium ions. Since the membrane is permeable to both Na^+ and K^+ this difference in concentration is not due to the ions being unable to pass through the membrane and establish equilibrium. Both ions do 'leak' across the membrane but the intracellular levels are maintained sensibly constant. Thus Na^+ must be 'pumped' out against a concentration gradient. Such a process which decreases the entropy or randomness of the system cannot occur spontaneously and energy must be provided to move the ions against the gradient. Furthermore the energy must be provided in a form such that it can be applied specifically to the ion that has to be moved. Such a specificity implies not only that the 'pumps' themselves must be specific for given ions and molecules, but also that they must be unidirectional.

Since the internal *milieu* of a cell is maintained more or less constant under conditions where the external medium is fluctuating widely there must be some sensing mechanism which governs the rate at which ions or molecules are pumped across the cell membrane. This is well illustrated by yeast cells which are able to survive changes in the culture medium from pH3 to pH10 – a ten millionfold change in H^+ concentration.

The metabolic energy required to power active transport processes is derived from glycolysis, respiration or adenosine triphosphate (ATP). In plants the last mentioned chemical is formed during photosynthetic phosphorylation – a complex reaction which utilises the light energy absorbed during the photosynthetic process. Subsequently the ATP is hydrolysed to form adenosine diphosphate (ADP) with the liberation of free energy. The actual mechanism by which this energy is used to actively transport the molecules across a cell membrane is enzymic. Enzymes are proteins which have the ability to catalyse chemical reactions and the difference in speed between an enzyme catalysed reaction and the corresponding non-enzymic reaction may well be in excess of a hundred millionfold. They are usually specific with respect to the reactions they can catalyse and the substrate that can be used.

Enzyme molecules are large compared with their substrate molecules and it follows that only a small part of the enzyme can be in contact with substrate. This area is called an active site and it is here that combination takes place during the formation of the enzyme – substrate complex. The presence of an active site imposes the necessity of correct orientation between enzyme and substrate before complex formation can occur. This is of little importance for reactions which take place in solution since the enzyme molecules are randomly arranged, but where enzymes are concerned with active transport processes they are actually built into the cell membrane. Under these conditions the enzyme molecule can only react with substrate on one side of the membrane and the requirement for unidirectional transport is satisfied (Fig. 6).

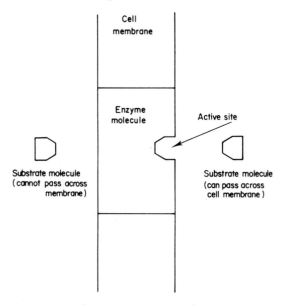

Fig. 6.—The enzyme molecule can only react with substrate on one side of the membrane.

It is possible for enzymes to be present as a mixture of active and inactive forms and the concentration of one relative to the other is determined partly by the genetical constitution of the cell. It follows that the rate of enzyme synthesis and its final concentration are part of the phenotypic expression of the cell and are therefore influenced by the intracellular environment.

One further factor which influences ion transport is the presence of a potential difference across the cell membrane. The inside of the cell is negative with respect to the outside and since natural membranes are extremely good insulators the potential difference can amount to well over 100mV. For example, in the alga *Nitella translucens* the potential difference between the outside of the cell and the cytoplasm is 140mV. Since the inside of the cell is negative the ingress of cations such as Na^+ will be assisted by an electrical force whereas anions such as $C1^-$ will not.

From this superficial look at the biological, biochemical and biophysical properties of cell membranes it would appear that their design was sufficiently sophisticated to enable them to maintain the *status quo* of the living cell irrespective of external conditions. This in fact is not true. It is possible to inhibit the active transport processes by the addition of certain chemicals to the external environment of the cell. When the heart drug ouabin is added to the tissues it inhibits the egress of Na^+ from the cells[17] Clearly if this happens the cell is unable to maintain the correct ionic composition. There is some evidence that the selective permeability of the cell membrane can be altered by a change in nutrition[18]. If the diet is low in unsaturated fatty acids new cell membranes and those being repaired may incorporate the wrong type of fat into the lipid layers. In crude terms this is rather like building or repairing a wall with bricks of the wrong shape or size. The resulting 'holes' will affect the permeability of the 'wall' or membrane. Sinclair attributes the lack of a correlation between smoking cigarettes and lung cancer found in Spain and Japan to the high level of unsaturated fatty acids found in diets of the people from those countries.

Obviously cell membranes are not perfect and if we return to our original question it seems likely that there will be a difference in the nutritional quality of food produced by the two methods of farming. Consider an ecosystem that over a period of time has been treated with biologically active sprays. Each of these chemicals has a definite half-life and one or more ways in which it will be degraded to other molecules, each of which has a half-life, etc. There will be present in the ecosystem small amounts of the active ingredients together with various residues and we have seen that it is possible for these to enter plant and animal cells. Apart from their biological activity there is the added factor that many of these compounds are man-made. Consequently plant and animal life will not have contacted them during evolution and there will be no natural biochemical pathways by which they are broken down into harmless substances. There will be no enzyme systems to degrade them and they will remain in the general metabolic pool of the plant or animal.

The possible teratogenic effect of the herbicide 2,4,5-T has recently received a great deal of publicity especially since this chemical, used as a defoliant, has been sprayed over vast areas in the Far East. There have been reports of women who subsequent to being in contact with the chemical have produced malformed babies. One is reminded of the thalidomide tragedy but there is one tremendous difference. Thalidomide was a drug specifically administered to humans and once the side effects were known it was immediately withdrawn from the market. 2,4,5-T on the other hand has been introduced non-specifically into an ecosystem. It can not be nullified nor can its half-life be accelerated and at this stage the long term biological effects can not be assessed.

References

1. Moore, N.W. (1969) *Biologist* 16, 157.
2. Mulder, D. (1953) Les elements mineurs en culture fruitière. 1^0 Convegno Nazionale di Frutticoltura, Montana di Saint Vincent, 188-198.
3. Bingham, F.T., and Garber, M.J. (1960) Solubility and availability of micronutrients in relation to phosphorous fertilization, *Soil Sci. Soc. Amer. Proc.* 24, 209-213.
4. Bingham, F.T., Martin, J.P., and Chastain, J.A. (1958) Effects of phosphorous fertilization of California soils on minor element nutrition of Citrus, *Soil Sci.* 86. 24-31.

5. Rogers, L.H., and Wu, C.H. (1948) Zinc uptake by oats as influenced by applications of lime and phosphate, *J. Amer. Soc. Agron.,* 40, 563-566.

6. Loneragan, J.F. (1951) The effect of applied phosphate on the uptake of zinc by flax, *Aust. J. Sci. Res. Ser. B.* 4, 108-114.

7. Chester, C.G.C. and Robinson, G.N. (1951) The role of zinc in plant metabolism, *Biol. Rev.* 26, 239-252.

8. Millikan, C.R. (1947) Effect of phosphates on the development of zinc deficiency symptoms in flax, *J. Dept. Agric. Victoria* 45, 273-278.

9. Stout, P.R., Meagher, W.R., Pearson, G.A. and Johnson, C.M. (1951) Molybdenum nutrition of crop plants. I. The influence of phosphate and sulphate on the absorption of molybdenum from soils and solution cultures. *Plant and Soils* 3, 51-87.

10. Ludwig, T.G., Healy, W.B. and Losee, F.L. (1960) An association between dental caries and certain soil conditions in New Zealand, *Nature,* 186, 695-696.

11. Ter Meulen, H. (1935) *Hand XXVe Ned. Natuurk. Geneesk. Congr.* 228.

12. Adler, P., and Straub, J. (1953) *Acta. Med. Acad. Sci. Hung.* 4, 221.

13. Nagy, Z., and Polyik, E. (1955) *Fogow. Syle.* 48, 154.

14. Legon, C.D. (1952) *Brit. Med. J.* ii, 700.

15. Griffith, G.W. (1960) *Soil and Cancer,* Medical Press, London.

16. Dittmer, H.J. (1949) Root-hair variations in plant species, *Amer. J. Bot.* 36, 152-155.

17. Marsden, J.C. (1970) Why do cells pump ions? *New Scientist* 22, 152-155.

18. Sinclair, H.M., see page 85 in this volume.

12. Soil microflora and basic nutritional concepts

A. Harry Walters, Fellow Inst. Biology, Fellow of Inst. Food Science and Technology and of The Royal Society of Health, Scientific Consultant to the Soil Association

Harry Walters believes that we should introduce the concept of probiotics in addition to antibiotics. Probiotics enlarge the concept of biological control and working with nature instead of against it.

IN 1967, at the annual Soil Association Conference, Professor Lindsay Robb said, 'The raw material of agriculture is life: we cannot create it and there is no substitute for it. Conserved and fostered within any biologically sound system of land use it is self-renewing all the time'. My interest is in the *kind* of life that was, is, and will be present in the soil.

Many years ago Dr. Hugh Nicol suggested that the principal natural raw materials of agriculture were soils and manures, both of which are directly or indirectly concerned with microbic life. So it might be said that microbes are basic to the life of the raw materials of agriculture. In the everyday world this fact is commonly overlooked because the farmer and gardener deals only with the final products of microbic production mechanisms which, primarily as soils, can be worked, handled and used for growing various forms of plant life for food, timber, drugs, decoration, oils or fibre, pulp and so on.

Everyone appreciates that with the aid of seed, sun, season and storm the soil is converted into plants, a process in which it is easy to recognise the parts played by other forms of life such as animals, birds, insects, worms and so on, since this can be seen with the naked eye, in part, if not wholly. But, in fact, by far the greatest contribution towards conversion from soil to plant is made by the microbes living and decaying in the earth, infinite billions of them which, of course, cannot be seen unless aided by the microscope. The part which these micro-organisms have played in the past, do now, and will play according to future trends in soil husbandry tends to be overlooked, forgotten, or just left to the expert.

A Moon's-Eye View

It is primarily in this role that I have been asked to relate soil micro-organisms to basic nutritional concepts. In order to put the subject into clear focus it might be useful in the first place to move off in the opposite direction and look at our planet briefly through the eyes of men who have journeyed to the moon and surveyed our globe from a distance of about a quarter of a million miles.

Astronaut Frank Borman said, 'Our earth is one hunk of ground, water, air and clouds floating around in space. From out there it is sure one world'. Jim Lovell said, 'The earth was the most beautiful thing there was to see in the heavens. People down there don't realise what they have. Up there it's a black-and-white world. There is no colour In the whole universe wherever we looked the only bit of colour was back on earth.' These most remarkable observers of our time looked at our earth in a manner similar to that of a microbiologist looking at a petri dish containing colonies of variously coloured bacteria, but in this case the substrate was that relatively exceedingly thin layer of rock, soil and water which is on the surface of the planet.

This tremendous human experience caused the three astronauts who were circumnavigating the moon at the end of 1968 to turn to basic philosophical concepts and broadcast a Christmas message to the world including the first ten verses of the Book of Genesis starting, 'In the beginning . . .'.

Nearer to home every one of us can see the fruits of this marvellous earth, but not many as yet appear to appreciate that the earth itself is alive physically, chemically, biochemically and biologically. This was the underlying theme of Lady Eve Balfour's book, *The Living Soil*[1], which led to the genesis of the Soil Association, and, linked to biophilosophical implications, the same applies to my book, *The Living Rocks*[2]. We are living in tremendous days because hitherto, from the historical angle, our view of this earth has been mainly subjective, since we have been too closely emotionally and possibly selfishly involved, But now that Man has got into space he can, for the first time in human history, take a moon's eye view of his own earth as a planet within the cosmos, and observe its uniqueness from a more objective, relatively detached angle. This means that once again he must start, 'In the beginning . . .'.

Microbes and the Genesis of the Soil

How did the soil on earth first arise and what part did microbes play in the process? Using the most modern and sophisticated techniques at present available the geochemists have put the age of this earth as a formed global structure between 4.8 and 5 thousand million years. Such figures are, of course, right outside human experience and dimension. Nevertheless, geological time can only be viewed in terms of the happenings which resulted in the formation of rock structures which are recognised today; periods during which mountain ranges, land masses, rivers, lakes, seas and glaciers formed and reformed; when all kinds of deposits and sediments as we know them today went through an amazing degree of processing under physical upheaval conditions which are quite beyond ordinary comprehension.

This fascinating historical concept is logged geologically through the Cainozoic period up to 50 million years back, then through the Mesozoic period which lasted about 150 million years, and the Palaeozoic period which goes back further some 300 million years, a total of 5-600 million years. Before that was the Precambrian period through which geological history recedes back and beyond for about another 4½ thousand million years when the earth, as mentioned, presumably assumed its global structure. Dr. Carol Alley, a physicist from Maryland University, said recently, 'Ever since Einstein it has been recognised that there is no common universal time.' Between the geochemists rushing us backwards through geological 'time', and the astronauts pushing us forward through cosmological 'time', this thing of 'time' is beginning to show many facets.

Examinations of sulphur isotopes in mineral deposits laid down some 800 million years ago give clear evidence of early activity of sulphur bacteria. Older still samples of rock taken from the Gunflint chert in Canada have an estimated age of over 2 thousand million years, and these were found to contain striking microscopical formations resembling blue-green algae and possibly thermophilic flexibacteria. These blue-green algae are closely related to the photosynthetic bacteria which utilise chlorophyll, while the thermophiles are heat-loving organisms. Those who have visited the natural thermal areas in Yellowstone Park, USA, and at Rotorua, New Zealand, which, in many respects, are probably quite near to very early conditions here on earth, where the atmosphere is still full of a sulphurous stench and steam, will be interested to learn that under such conditions microbes have been isolated capable of growing at near boiling point. These are the only forms of biological life in the immediate vicinity of the geysers, boiling mud pools and the like.

Since, in the very early times, there was no free oxygen in the biosphere, these pioneers of biological life as unicellular forms, were almost certainly anaerobic or anoxygenic and waterborne. They appear first to have shown up during the period when there was sedimentation of the earth's crust and secondary substances and conditions appeared capable of supporting biological life. From the Palaeozoic era onwards there is a well-documented record

M

of fossils and other geological specimens related not only to single-celled microbes but also to chlorophyll-containing plants and Metazoa in general which are multicellular.

From these concepts of the world's early history, in which Man played no part at all, it can be seen that primitive metabolism must have been continually reaching some kind of balance with the immense physical, chemical and pre- and post-biochemical changes which were taking place at the period. Under such dynamic conditions there probably were no clear divisions between the various kinds of activities taking place.

For instance, the parts played, not only by the various sulphur compounds and other types of inorganic and organic chemical conjugations, but also that of the different forms of Precambrian iron sedimentation and other minerals, must have been most important during this flux of conversion, transmutation and adaptation. Under such early earth conditions water would have protected simple biological life from any adverse effects of direct UV irradiation and also from any toxic concentrations of gases in the lower layers of the earth's atmosphere. In fact, one branch of geochemistry now deals – relative to the conditions operating in the beginning – with the study of the formation of mineralised organic substances and the importance of micro-organisms and their decomposition products in the migration of chemical elements.

The Gigantic Compost

It is now perhaps permissible to view the genesis of the soil in terms of the world's prehistory partly as a fabulous and gigantic composting operation, which led to sedimentation of various kinds. Indeed, the role of living organisms, their metabolic products and detritus, and the salts of seawater, are all linked together in a chain of events which are connected with bacterial activity relative to such sediment formation. At quite an early stage, biochemical conversion of all types of organic matter was involved, but here there were great differences in origin, formation, and conditions of burial and decomposition. Many polymeric compounds were broken down and utilised by living organisms, while monomeric compounds participated in secondary reactions leading to the formation of substances such as humic acids and melanoidins which are present in the basic composition of soil, peat and coal.

The products of living organism decomposition at various stages in their conversion to mineralised organic compounds were also incorporated into such widely differing sedimented substances as petroleum, shale oil, amber, saltpetre, organic acids, pigments, phenolics, proteins, amino acids and lipids. The degradation of protein to amino acids is stepwise due to progressive enzymatic action, and polypeptides and amino acids can be detected in soils, sediments, plankton and natural waters.

Sediments taken from the Pacific Ocean at depths between 30-7,500 metres have been found to contain substances such as chlorophyll and carotene, and carotenoids have been isolated from natural water deposits known to be at least 20,000 years old. So it is possible to link the primaeval decomposition of organic matter from all kinds of biological vegetation to animals, birds, fish and micro-organisms in oceans, lakes and rivers, with the formation of many organic deposits, suspensions and solutions on the earth's crust.

Commenting on the significance of degradative products of proteins, carbohydrates, fats and pigments, Vernadsky, the Russian authority, has suggested that the basic process appears to have been that organisms died under water under anaerobic conditions and formed immense concentrations of decomposition products, and that on this substrate the early mass of living material was over-flowing with bacteria and possibly fungi. Enormous masses of living organisms participated in the formation of limestone, sandstone and other rocks, the organic parts of the decaying organisms being decomposed while the mineral constituents were preserved in the rocks.

It would appear that up to the Ordovician era around 300-350 million years ago (Palaeozoic), it was marine life which fulfilled the most important role relative to sedimentation. Later, however, following the transition of biological life from water on to the land, particularly in the Cainozoic era around 50 million years ago, sedimentary accumulations developed in coastal bogs and flood plains where bryophytic coals came into being. It has now been established that in the coalification process the activity of algae, fungi and bacteria together with the degradation products of plants, animals, insects, amphibia, reptiles and fish have all been involved.

When one considers how deep into the earth's surface the known deposits have been traced so far, and the immense biologically degradative and chemically transmutative processes which have taken place, it is then that the living soil becomes a vividly animate entity, which merits the closest possible study of all the life it contains in every form in order to preserve and encourage its fertility. Biophilosophically speaking, it may have now become obvious why I wrote in *The Living Rocks* that 'From the modern standpoint, one of the most arresting features of the story of the Creation (Genesis, 1) is the sequence in which the events are recorded... heaven, earth, light, night, day, water, land, plant-life and the seed-bearing cycle, the seasons, the years, the sun, moon and stars, and the creatures of the sea, the air ... and the land.'

Prolife Concepts and Microbial Balance in Soil

Having traced something of the historical aspects, it is quite clear that the living soil has always been a living entity from every scientific point of view, and that microorganisms from the outset have played a very significant part. Although today, soil microbiology is a highly developed science, I suggest that it can no longer be thought of as being an activity confined to just a few experts, but rather that all its aspects should become more widely appreciated and understood.

In this respect perhaps some kind of parallel might be drawn with the study of medicine. About a century ago the microbic basis for infectious disease was discovered, but it was not until fifty or more years later that the true significance of this discovery was beginning to be appreciated outside medical circles. Even within medical circles acceptance of it was by no means immediate, and, as late as 1906, Shaw, in his play *The Doctor's Dilemma* was still laughing at the idea of 'stimulating the phagocytes' to fight invading germs. In 1848, before the discoveries of Pasteur, Semmelweis had demonstrated that washing the hands in hypochlorite as a disinfectant could dramatically control the incidence of puerperal fever in maternity hospitals. This still goes on today in the form of washing cows udders for the control of spread of mastitis.

Following on the work of Semmelweis, Pasteur, Lister, Koch and others, the idea of achieving chemical control of microbic infection caught the chemists' imagination, and the first great breakthrough was made in 1908 by Ehrlich with arsanil, which went on until 1935 when Domagh first described sulphonamide. The whole concept of chemotherapy was *'anti'*-infection. Although it is still valuable in certain conditions its main function was almost entirely replaced by the advent of penicillin through Fleming, Florey and Chain in 1940. Despite the fact that penicillin was the product of a living organism, since it prevented the proliferation of harmful microbes in the human body, initially it was called an *'anti'*-biotic, in other words the biological equivalent of a chemical anti-infection agent.

From a biophilosophical viewpoint it would have perhaps been more apt to call penicillin a *Pro*biotic, inasmuch as it is the product naturally associated with symbiotic control and could not harm the host. It is interesting to note that 25 years after the discovery of penicillin, a paper appeared by Drs. Lilley and Stillwell called 'Probiotics – Growth-Promoting Factors produced by Micro-organisms', yet when penicillin was included in animal and bird feeding stuffs for the purpose of promoting growth in the host it was still called an *anti*biotic! Hence, although the prefix 'anti' was inherited directly from its chemical precursors, on the evidence I have presented, from Sammelweis to Fleming, the advent of antibiotics might be considered as a scientific progression through chemical germicides, disinfectants, antiseptics and specific chemotherapeutic agents on to a biological *Pro*duct, which, within very wide limits of applications, has proved relatively harmless to the host indicating its *Pro*biotic proclivities. In other words, the approach is to engender a state of healthy biological balance, a biophilosophical condition which I described in a chapter entitled 'Prolife and Antilife' in my book already mentioned.

In the field of soil and animal husbandry I feel that some similar kind of progression of events is in train, that is, from chemical treatments to probiotics. In order to remedy certain deficiencies in the soil, additions of suitable chemical fertiliser and mineral formulations have been found of inestimable value. It has also been found that such formulations can increase production from already adequately fertile soils, and, at present, this discovery is being exploited to the uttermost. In some cases it has now reached the point of over-exploitation and a wide variety of obvious side-effects are now becoming apparent ranging from pollution of water supplies to over-production and exhaustion.

A number of perhaps not-so-obvious side-effects may also be appearing. For instance, recently while engaged on a haematological investigation in a maternity hospital, I observed that in a series of two thousand patients, many women who subsisted mainly on forced-fertilised and variously-processed or frozen foods showed an increased incidence of anaemia during pregnancy. Subsequent tests taken on such women, particularly immigrants and women at work, showed diminished blood serum iron, vitamin B_{12} and folic acid levels, but treatment with iron invariably resulted in a dramatic increase to normal haemoglobin levels.

In debilitated underfed populations, (outside the effects of worm infestations) the link between faulty nutrition and anaemia together with certain idiopathic diarrhoeic conditions has long been known. In the nineteenth century, during the rapid rise of the Industrial Revolution when human populations left the land and were herded into towns to live, work and breed often on poor food, anaemias were very common, and some of the most popular 'tonics' of those times were based on iron compounds. Special types of primary chlorotic anaemias were usually blamed onto too tight lacing of corsets, but even these patients usually responded well to dietary supplements of liver and iron.

Today, there is a striking parallel. Animals are being taken off the land and herded into what I call the equivalents of 'animal towns' (with apologies to George Orwell) for rearing. Under such artificial conditions often anaemia and scouring results, so much so that the administration of iron compounds, chemically prepared, and other drugs has now become routine. For instance, despite the fact that pigs and piglets are now widely reared in hygienic concrete houses, anaemia and scouring are far more to be feared than ever they were with free-range pigs.

This appears to indicate that the conditions of life in modern 'animal towns' are such that essential Prolife ingredients are missing, and the animal gut, as a microbial conversion factory – a biochemical unit – cannot supply the necessary metabolic requirements sufficiently balanced in a form that can be readily osmosed through the gut wall. In fact, I suspect that in some cases there might even be a reverse osmosis going on whereby essential metabolites are reintroduced from the blood stream into the gut causing essential nutrient losses.

Research Toward an Ordered Economy

It seems to me that the whole matter is one of maintaining a balance, and the more naturally that balance can be achieved according to Prolife concepts the better results are likely to be in the long term. This applies to every aspects of growing food, and includes the necessary balance of requisite types and numbers of macro- and micro-organisms within the soil itself and also in manures employed according to location and use to which the land is put. It must also apply to those tending the soil, for them to regard it as a living entity in itself, as already mentioned, and the more they know about soil microbiology from Winogradsky (1889) onwards perhaps the better, and the more totally fruitful the soil is likely to be. That is what Professor Robb meant when he stressed the importance of understanding self-renewal of the land.

It has been made abundantly clear that substances considered absolutely essential for human and animal nutrition such as carbohydrates, proteins, fats, minerals, pigments and so on, all originally came into being in prehistoric times by processes which were intimately linked with active microbic action. I believe that the part which a wider knowledge of microbic response to soil husbandry can play is potentially immense. The present era of mainly chemical treatment is now at its peak, a position from which farming eventually must move on. I look forward in the future to quite exciting advances in Prolife fundamentals in our knowledge of the utilisation of soil micro-organisms in basic nutritional concepts.

To obtain truly worthwhile advances I think the scientific endeavour must be linked to an overall biophilosophy. I first coined this term in 1967, and it is interesting to observe that in September of the next year (1968) a whole section of the international meeting of the Vitalstoffgesell-schaft held in Hanover on Diseases of Civilisation was devoted to 'Biophilosophical Reflections on Life Processes on the Basis of the Exact Natural Sciences' – to which no less than six professors from various continental universities contributed papers.

The research now developing in the Soil Association at Haughley is following this lead and looking to the future with confidence. There are now sufficient indications that the next step forward will rest on advancing on the natural raw materials of agriculture as soils and manures regarded as living Probiotics, and experiments now being planned in this direction should certainly show promising results.

Together with the scientific aspects, I have also stressed the importance of the biophilosophical side so perhaps it might be best if I closed on a remark of Epictetus, Roman philosopher of the early days of the Piscean Age some 2,000 years ago who wrote that 'reaping of corn means the destruction of the ears, but this is not evil, neither is the fall of the leaf, nor that the green fig should be dried, nor that raisins should be made from grapes: All these are changes from a former state into another, not for destruction but an ordered economy'. And set this beside the observation made by Astronaut Lovell at the close of the Piscean Age, 'The earth was the most beautiful thing there was to see in the heavens. People down there don't realise what they have'.

References

1. *The Living Soil,* Faber and Faber, London, 1943.
2. *The Living Rocks,* Classic Publications. London, 1967.

13. Preliminary considerations and the methods used in the investigations of nutritional values at the Soil Association Research Farms

D.B. Long, M.A., Ph.D., Director, Michaelis Nutritional Research Laboratory, Harpenden

The contributors to this symposium have all shown the new threats to the health of western man that arise from his diet as a result of his technological triumphs both in growing and processing food. In this article Dr. Long outlines some of the research that could be done into the nutritional value of food according to the way it is grown. He points out that the Soil Association's Research Farms can provide the ideal material. What is required is the funds from outside sources to make this essential research possible.

UNDERLYING the work of the Soil Association is the concept that the state of health in man may at least in part be traced back through animal products and crops to the state of the soil from which his food originated. The first really practical contribution came with the policy governing the setting up of the Haughley Experiment. This, amongst other points, provided for the study of changes in soil condition and chemistry and also a study of quality in produce, all resulting from the use of three different farming methods. Thus, an 'organic' method, using only naturally occurring processes, could be contrasted with current farming practice, using artificial fertilisers either with or without the involvement of animals on two separate sections termed 'mixed' and 'stockless' respectively.

For purposes of growth, most plants obtain their energy from sunlight and, apart from carbon dioxide which is absorbed from the air, they are generally entirely dependent on soil for their supply of water and nutrient substances. It might be expected that the organic method would lead to a build-up of a soil rich in naturally occurring organic material and soil fauna, which would provide the best environment for healthy plant growth by making available the widest possible range of plant nutrients, together with the best physical conditions for root development and water uptake. In contrast, it might be expected that, by introducing through the use of artificial fertilisers a very restricted range of plant nutrients, nitrogen, phosphate and potassium (NPK), a previously established biological system would be disturbed in such a way as to reduce the availability and possibly the range of other nutrients and ultimately to affect the physical state of the soil, thus producing an inferior plant and crop. This presents a fundamental problem which, because of its complexity and ever-present economic pressures, has never been scientifically resolved, despite its great importance to the well-being of mankind. The Soil Association has taken up this problem and over recent years has set itself increasingly to the task of scientifically establishing the truth of the situation as it actually occurs in the field on its experimental farms.

Before looking at methods that are being developed to attack this task, some of the inherent complexity of the problem must be appreciated.

Soil

Soil itself is not a uniform substance but is heterogenous – that is, it is a mixture both physical and chemical. For example:

(a) Its particle size can vary from minute crystals and fragments, as in silts and clays, to large stones and rocks.

(b) The mineral composition varies according to the particular type of rock from which it was formed, as can be seen by contrasting the red soil in Devon formed from red sandstone with the pale calcareous soils of Kent based on chalk and limestones.

(c) The organic content, such as the humus of rich loams, the fibre of peaty soils and the protein of heavy clays, affect its physical nature and the potential of chemical quality.

(d) Soil is not just an inert substance but it is an inter-related biological complex containing a living fauna of bacteria and many lower forms of life.

(e) Normally the composition is highly variable, both from area to area and from season to season, being subject to the disturbances of cultivation, crop root growth, the movements and changes in its living population. and the leaching effects of rain.

In such a study the nutrient elements are of vital importance. Broadly speaking they can be divided into two groups:

Major or Macro elements which form the bulk of plant material and, apart from carbon, hydrogen and oxygen, include:

Nitrogen	Phosphorus	Potassium
Calcium	Magnesium	Sulphur

Minor or Trace elements which form only a minute part of plant material, some being present in as low as one part in several million and which include:

Iron	Zinc	Copper
Manganese	Molybdenum	Cobalt
Sulphur	Boron	Iodine

In general, the major elements are incorporated directly in plant tissues, whereas the minor elements, together with certain major elements, are intimately involved with enzyme systems, either as part of the enzyme molecule itself or as activators which must be present for enzyme function. Fully functional enzyme systems are essential for life as they govern all the life processes including the vitality of the plant and its growth rate. Throughout this century much attention has been given to the tissue building elements of nitrogen, phosphorus and potassium (NPK), together with calcium (lime) which indeed must be present in adequate quantities for vigorous plant growth. The truth of this has led to the rapid development of the artificial fertiliser industry with its high rate concentrates, but it is only more recently that attention is being given to some of the other elements which are automatically excluded from modern highly-purified fertilisers.

The effectiveness of NPK has established the law of minimum quantities so that it would appear to be a simple matter to embrace the whole range of nutrients in an ideal artificial fertiliser that ensured that there would be a minimum quantity of each essential element present. However, if such an artificial fertiliser were ever to be produced and set before the public as the perfect plant nutrient fertiliser, the claim would be false because:

1. Some elements are more soluble and mobile than others and are more easily leached out by rain. Thus, at any one time, apart from the effect of soil type, the proportions of the various elements supplied by the fertiliser will vary according to the time elapsed since application, the rainfall, soil drainage rate, and the depth of soil sample.

2. Different types of soil adsorb onto the surface of soil particles different amounts of the various elements and not necessarily in the proportions that these elements were supplied. Sandy soils generally adsorb least and soils with a high organic or protein content (e.g. clay) most elements. Subsequently certain of these adsorbed elements may be progressively released as they are exchanged for others. Furthermore, in this process previously contained elements may be released also so that completely different amounts from those in the original fertiliser may ultimately be available to the plant. Within this context, the pH, that is the acidity or alkalinity of the soil, is extremely important. Some elements, such as iron, manganese, copper and zinc, are only soluble and

mobile in acid media, whereas other elements, such as molybdenum and calcium, are more freely available in alkaline soils. Thus, the soil pH strongly influences the nutrient elements that may ultimately be actually available to the plant.

3. The various elements interact with each other affecting the availability and usefulness to particular plants. Generally the effect is one of antagonism as, for example, that of high levels of soil phosphorus which will interfere with copper, zinc, potassium and iron uptake or utilisation which may thus induce deficiencies of these four elements.

Other examples of antagonism are:
Nitrogen on potassium and boron.
Zinc on iron.
Magnesium on potassium.
Copper on iron and manganese.
Calcium on zinc, boron, magnesium, potassium and manganese.
Manganese on iron.

From the above it can be seen that it should be possible to apply to soil large amounts of sewage sludge which has a high zinc content without producing toxic symptoms provided adequate quantities of calcium (lime) are also added to antagonise the zinc, and this has been experimentally established elsewhere. At the same time, care must be taken that induced deficiencies of boron, magnesium, potassium or manganese do not simultaneously develop. A few elements interact in such a way as to enhance the effect of others. Such effects exist between:
Phosphorus on magnesium
Nitrogen on magnesium
Potassium on manganese and iron

Thus it can be seen that a limiting factor in plant growth cannot be simply determined as a deficiency in the minimum requirement of a specific plant nutrient. The Law of the Maximum must also be applied, namely that the nutrient present in the relative maximum also determines the yield. The widespread injudicious use of fertilisers in current times has led to many unexplained reductions in yield due to induced deficiencies, and this needs to be constantly borne in mind when considering the nutritional value of soil under different methods of husbandry.

Plants

A primary difficulty in the use of crops for assessment is that weight is the generally accepted parameter. As plants are seldom grown under optimum conditions, extra stimulation of the growth potential will increase weight, but this is not necessarily related to a balanced state of plant development. The excessive use of sugars and starches in the diet of man may lead to extra growth in the formation of fatty tissue, but this would not normally be regarded as balanced growth and desirable. Thus the criteria for assessing balanced growth in plants or crops needs to be more specifically defined.

Balanced growth would presumably occur in soils presenting a balanced nutrition and, from what has been previously stated on the inter-relationships of nutrients, balanced nutrition can occur throughout a whole range of levels for individual nutrients from the minimum required to the maximum tolerated. However, further complexities may exist here if the hypothesis of C.L. Kervran proves correct, in which he proposes that plants, amongst other forms of life, convert certain elements into others, particularly if they are present in excess.

Such a proposal is quite outside our present knowledge of classical chemistry, the only elemental transmutations known being in the realm of atomic science. This, therefore, demands further attention. The proposition is based on the fact that throughout the biological world there are instances when quantitatively the chemical composition does not appear to be related to the substrate composition. For example, magnesium in sea water is considered to be transformed in the presence of oxygen into calcium by

181

crustaceans (crabs, lobsters, etc.), calcareous seaweeds, corals, etc., because the organism ultimately contains more of this element than can be accounted for in the original substrate. This is also thought to take place in germinating seedlings and, if true, demonstrates the importance of the correct balance between magnesium and calcium in the soil, although Professor Kervran has pointed out that not all plants have this capacity and such plants, must, therefore have adequate calcium in the soil. Similar conversions are considered to take place in animals where, for example, potassium or silicate can be changed into calcium in chicken eggshell formation and, in the case of men working in the Sahara, more magnesium has been found to be excreted than can be accounted for in their food and drink, whereas there appears to be a deficit of sodium.

Thus, it can be seen that a plant may not simply reflect the availability of its contained elements and considerable work and care must be made in the interpretation of results. If the views of Professor Kervran ultimately prove to be true, the whole fundamental basis of existing knowledge of soil fertility will have to be systematically reviewed.

Methods Used

The basic methods of scientific approach to the problem fall under one or more of the following:
1. Direct analytical study of soil fertility.
2. Plant or crop assay of soil fertility.
3. Animal assays.

1. *Soil Analyses*
A total analysis of the nutrients present in soil has little meaning within the context of the experiment, because many nutrients may be 'locked away' by interaction with other substances in the soil and thus be unavailable to the growing plant. Over the years much attention has been given to this problem of how the nutrients actually available

can best be determined. More recently it has been found that by leaching with a neutral salt solution – that is one which is neither acidic or alkaline – reproducible results can be obtained which make reliable comparisons possible.

However, the heterogenous nature of soil, with its great variability, presents a further big problem in the reproducibility required for scientific analyses. At Rothamsted, experiments showed that, for a meaningful comparison of experimental plots, it was necessary to take soil samples not more than three feet apart in any direction, resulting in thousands of samples for multiple plot experiments. In a systematic area survey on a field approximately 350 x 250 yd. the phosphorus content varied in different zones from 1 to 14mg per 100g of soil. Similar zonal variations have been observed in the growth of crops and distribution of grazing animals which can be related to zonal differences in the nutritional composition of the soil. From this, it is apparent that attempts to relate total crop yields and analyses from a given field to random soil samples can be quite meaningless and only by working on analytically surveyed areas can this difficulty be minimised.

Physical properties such as humus, water-holding capacity and pH, together with chemical composition such as NPK, can be determined relatively easily in the laboratory, but, with such large numbers of samples, an auto-analyser, which simultaneously analyses for a number of factors on an automated conveyor-belt principle handling up to seventy samples an hour, must be used. The analysis of minerals, including trace elements, however, has in the past been a lengthy and sometimes complicated matter, involving chemical separation and production of a coloured metallic salt or complex which in solution could be measured spectrophotometrically – that is, by measuring the intensity of coloured light of the appropriate wavelength passed through the solution from a constant light source and comparing it with that which passed through a standard solution. The analysis of certain elements takes an appreciable time and this drastically restricts the number of samples handled. The recent development of physical methods of analysis, such as atomic absorption, to the levels of sensitivity needed for soil and crop analysis, makes possible an entirely new approach requiring multiple analyses.

For the benefit of those to whom atomic absorption is an unfamiliar if not awe-inspiring name, a few words follow on the principles involved. Atomic absorption is a development of a complementary character to flame photometry. In this, the sample in solution form is sprayed into a gas/air flame where alkali metals and other volatile elements are converted into a vapour made of atoms of the elements present. Some of the atoms absorb heat energy from the flame and ionise, emitting a characteristic wavelength of light (rather like a sodium lamp) as they return to the unexcited 'ground' state. The intensity of this light is directly proportional to the concentration of material present and can be measured photometrically.

Obviously this technique is restricted to the few volatile elements. The remainder, however, can be handled by atomic absorption as, with a suitable flame, an atomic vapour in the unexcited ground state can be produced from the sample. If then light of the wavelength appropriate to the element being analysed is projected through this vapour, an amount of light will be absorbed by the vapour proportional to the concentration of the element present and, with the use of a suitable wavelength isolation device to cut out other extraneous wavelengths, the decrease in intensity can be measured photometrically. Lamps are used producing exactly the right light wavelengths by having a cathode of the element to be analysed. Such an instrument can analyse samples up to one hundred per hour for each element, and other elements can be selected by changing the lamp and wavelength of the absorption line.

Returning to the soil, it is apparent that the mode of action of NPK in stimulating plant growth is still uncertain. With regard to nitrogen, it has been pointed out that only a small percentage of that applied is taken up directly by the plant, whilst soil analyses have shown that, after an application, it disappears quite rapidly. Part, at least, of the nitrogen is leached out by rainfall and drains into lakes and rivers as has been shown by Professor Commoner and others, but the fate of even these three basic nutrients in the soil needs to be more fully understood.

It has been realised that the microflora (bacteria and other soil organisms) of soil may not only affect the availability of plant nutrients but also synthesise various substances which affect the plant itself and the nutritional value to mankind of the ensuing crop. The soil fauna will inevitably need a minimum supply of organic material containing potential nutrients for its own maintenance, so that limited applications of compost can be too small for this purpose. In such cases, extra applications of compost will not just stimulate plant growth and increase crop yields but will basically affect the nature and extent of the development of the bacterial flora. On the other hand, applications of fertilisers which ignore this requirement will almost certainly change the nature of the bacterial flora and the extent of its role in plant nutrition.

From this, it is apparent that serious attention should be given to the suggestion that a new approach be made at Haughley to this problem of the effect of fertilisers on soil, in which continuous parallel studies are made of changes in bacterial flora and the availability of plant nutrients. To study this, relatively small plots need to be marked off in selected fields so that a realistic number of samples can be taken at frequent and regular intervals. The relationship between bacterial flora and the presence of plant nutrients could then be studied and, as this fundamental relationship became understood, attention given to the problem of crop growth in relation to the nutritional and biological state of the soil. It must be stressed, however, that this is no small task. Rothamsted has worked on aspects of this problem for over fifty years and only now, with recent technological advances, is it beginning to make progress. Thus, for Haughley, such a project cannot be accomplished at little cost by a few soil samples taken over a few months but must be viewed as one which will require adequate financial provision for the full assistance of modern auto-mated systems and, once started, would need to continue for a number of years to cover all the variables involved. Such important research, therefore, will almost inevitably depend upon the willingness of grant-aiding bodies such as the A.R.C. to assist but, unfortunately, no help of any kind has so far been forthcoming, despite the unusual value of the experimental material and the unique experimental possibilities this presents.

Mr. J.F. Ward, in his summary on analyses in the Haughley Experiment for the years 1952-1956, points out factors which suggest a decline in soil fertility on the organic section. During that period, in the course of a ten-year rotation, there were two applications of 10-12 tons per acre of compost on the organic, whereas the mixed section received 24-30 tons of F.Y.M. and 32-36 cwt. of fertiliser, apart from slag. What has been achieved on the organic section is remarkable but this raises the question as to whether the quantities of compost and the number of applications were, in fact, adequate. The concern here is, of course, the biological implications of this problem along the lines previously indicated. The correct applications to maintain a balanced nutrition and high level of fertility could best be determined by relating a soil analysis to the new wealth of information that this proposed experimental method would produce.

2. Plant or Crop Assays

No experimental work has been developed to assay soil fertility by observations on plant material in the period covered by this report.

3. Animal Assays

Although the ultimate in crop and animal product assay lies in nutrition studies in man, initial work can be profitably carried out with animals where the environment is more uniform or can be more easily controlled. A report has been prepared on the Small Animal Feeding Experiment which makes it clear that even the controlling of the animal environment is not all that simple.

Apart from the Small Animal Feeding Experiment, the farm animals available for nutritional assay are cows and chicken. Much attention has already been drawn to milk production in cows in which the organic cows give more milk per pound of food than the mixed. Apart from this, unfortunately, their numbers are too small for rapid decisive results owing to considerably individual variation including differences in the age structure of the two herds. Nevertheless, as part of the study of the biology of the cow, which includes lactation performance, calving and general health, the haematology and chemistry of the blood was also studied. There was a definite suggestion that the 'mixed' herd was more restless than the 'organic' and there were significant differences in the fatty composition of the bloods of the two herds, a finding which could prove to be of singular importance in view of the role of such fatty substances in the incidence of coronary diseases.

Assays with sheep in the past suffered similar limitations to those with cows; numbers were still too small for definite conclusions to be drawn with confidence on a single year's observation. However, differences were found similar to those in cows in respect of the suggestion of a greater restlessness in the 'mixed' flock and also in the fatty composition of the sheep blood. Differences were also observed in the cellular composition of the bloods of the two flocks which suggested that the 'mixed' flock had blood with a greater oxygen carrying capacity which may have reflected a greater basic oxygen requirement in these sheep. As part of the sheep assay, wool samples were also studied and differences found between the flocks. The indication has been that organic feeding does not produce the finest quality wool as assessed by the Wool Marketing Board as quality is determined in terms of fineness of the fibre rather than regularity and strength, and fine wool is generally produced by weaker or more sickly sheep.

'Organic' sheep produce wool which is sounder with fewer thin or short staples, although slightly less uniform than the 'mixed' wool.

Chicken, on the other hand, offer a sufficient supply of genetically homozygous material to provide statistically valuable data that could give a conclusive answer to the dietetic effect of crop husbandry. At Haughley, chicken are kept under ideal free-range conditions where, by their own efforts, birds on organic or mixed pastures can still make good possible deficiencies. However, the majority of modern eggs are produced by battery systems where differences between diets based on organically produced crops and those produced with artificial fertilisers would best be revealed. Ideally a four treatment experiment could be set up and has been planned accordingly.

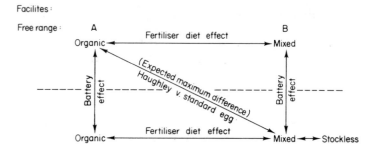

The experiment should be set up from an organic homozygous chicken source to minimise variety variations with about 150 birds in each group. Two groups of birds would be kept under normal free range conditions on organic (A) and mixed (B) diets at Haughley. The remaining three groups of birds would be kept under battery conditions: their feeding stuffs would be taken from the organic (C) mixed (D) and stockless (E) sections, comparable supplies of organic and mixed feeding stuffs being given to both the free range and battery birds. Observations would be made on growth and maturation, fecundity or egg-laying rate of the birds with routine blood and feather analyses and finally tissue studies including flavour tests. The use of modern ultra-micro equipment permits multiple analyses on small quantities of blood and thus does not require the death of birds. Tests on the eggs would include observations on viability and weight of hatchings, grade, egg faults, egg analysis (including trace elements and lipids), shell strength and flavour tests.

Such an experiment would scientifically contrast the produce from an organic free-range poultry farm with that from standard battery systems by comparing A with D and E. This then can be broken down to show the effect of the 'fertiliser' diet by contrasting B with A for free range and D and E with C for battery conditions. The actual effect of battery conditions would be shown by contrasting C with A and D with B. This naturally would apply to both eggs and birds and, apart from establishing any superiority of organic foods, would also provide other fundamental information for the poultry farmer on the comparative merits of the different diets and systems.

This experiment is, of course, expressed in the ideal form and many modifications of the layout are possible whereby chicken could be most usefully used to assay the nutritional value of organic foods.

Summary

With the development of modern technology and the comparatively recent availability of automated apparatus, more new detailed approaches are possible to the basic methods of investigation in the Haughley Experiment which may be listed:

1. A direct analytical study of soil fertility.
2. Plant and crop assays of soil fertility.
3. Animal assays.

In direct analytical studies of fertility, the part played by the microbiology of the soil and its relationship to soil chemistry should now be considered so that the effect of application of fertilisers is both more fully understood and scientifically demonstrated. Such techniques, too, make it possible to establish in crop and animal assays a meaningful relationship with soil fertility, in terms of ultimate nutritional value. However, as with the proposed direct study of soil fertility, sufficient financial support to implement the chicken assay experiment has also not been available. Thus it can be seen that, with these scientific developments, the range of experiments that can be made on material derived from Haughley in the nutritional field is very wide indeed and limited now only by financial consideration.

INDEX

Index